WOMEN, AIDS, & COMMUNITIES

A Guide for Action

by
Gerry Pearlberg

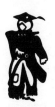

Women's Action Alliance, Inc.
and
The Scarecrow Press, Inc.
Metuchen, N.J., & London

WOMEN'S ACTION ALLIANCE, INC.

Founded in 1971, the Alliance is a national organization committed to furthering the goal of full equality for all women. We work towards this end by providing educational programs and services that assist women and women's organizations in accomplishing their goals.

Women, AIDS, & Communities: A Guide for Action was developed for the Women's Centers and AIDS Project at Women's Action Alliance, Inc. Content is solely the responsibility of Women's Action Alliance, Inc., 370 Lexington Avenue, Suite 603, New York, NY 10017.

British Library Cataloguing-in-Publication data available.

Library of Congress Cataloging-in-Publication Data

Pearlberg, Gerry.
    Women, AIDS, & communities : a guide for action / by Gerry Pearlberg.
        p.   cm.
    Includes bibliographical references and index.
    Cloth ISBN 0-8108-2470-1 (alk. paper)
    Paper ISBN 0-8108-2450-7 (alk. paper)
    1. AIDS (Disease)--Social aspects. 2. Women--Diseases.
3. Women's health services. 4. Community health services.
I. Title. II. Title: Women, AIDS, and communities.
RA644.A25P42 1991
362.1'969792'0082--dc20   91-17428

I wish to dedicate this book to the memory of M. Brooks Jones, 1944-1989. Remembering him is a sad and frequent reminder to me of what this epidemic means in personal terms and why it must be stopped.

Contents

Contents

Acknowledgments

This guidebook would not have been possible without the personal support and practical assistance of the many friends, colleagues, and women's centers' staff members with whom I had the honor of working during my time as the director of the Women's Centers and AIDS Project and since. It is a pleasure to acknowledge them here.

I would like to express my appreciation to those persons involved in women's issues and in AIDS prevention, activism, and service delivery who generously reviewed and commented at various stages of the manuscript: Joan Altman, Alexis Danzig, Sharen Duke, Nicholas Freudenberg, Lynnette Gosch, Elissa Greene, Jennifer Gunnell, Linda Gutterman, Gail Harris, Joyce Klemperer, Frances Kunreuther, Rebecca Porper, Hernan Poza III, Luisa Mesquita, Dagmar Santiago, Edith Springer, Barbara Stanley, and Heather Stephenson.

The Women's Centers and AIDS Project's Advisory Board gave considerable support during the process of developing this book. In particular, I wish to thank Lynne McArthur, Denise Ribble, Wendy Chavkin, and Joanne Mantell for their generous assistance.

Many thanks to Women's Action Alliance's former Executive Director Sylvia Kramer for her support of this project, and to the following staff members for providing technical assistance and guidance: Elizabeth Lopez, Tracey McDougall, Mary McGinnis, Judy Rowley, Christie Timms, and Dominique Treboux. Linda Campbell, who took the reigns of the Women's Centers and AIDS Project after my departure, provided help and encouragement at a particularly critical point in the process of completing this project.

In my current position at the New York City Department of Health, I have benefitted from the support and expertise of my wonderful friends and colleagues Matthew Frey and Elisabeth Tapley. I would also like to thank Beth Cohen and Lezli Redmond of the NYCDOH Library of AIDS Resources for their help in locating references and citations.

Ellen Leuchs deserves special recognition for her assistance and hard work through every stage of this effort. In her capacity both as the former Project Assistant for the Women's Centers and AIDS Project and as this book's editorial assistant, typist, and designer, she was always good humored, insightful, and helpful beyond the call of duty. I am grateful for her commitment to this project and for having had the opportunity to work with her.

The Women's Centers and AIDS Project (and this book) would not have been possible without the generous support of: Prudential Foundation, American Express Foundation, AT&T Foundation, Metropolitan Life Foundation, New York Community Trust, Fund for the City of New York, Xerox Corporation, Hoffman-LaRoche Foundation, Booth Ferris Foundation, DIFFA, New York State AIDS Institute, Morgan Guaranty Trust Co., Ms. Foundation for Women, Pettus Crowe Foundation, Living Arts Foundation, and the United Way.

Introduction

This book is intended to encourage service providers and advocates at women's centers and other community-based organizations (CBOs) to become involved in providing AIDS-related services, information, and education for women. We believe that organizations such as yours are appropriate and important agents for increasing awareness about women and AIDS, and for advocating that greater resources be directed toward prevention and services for underserved women and families. This guide is designed to provide an overview of the information, resources, and support you will need to begin to do this vital work.

The epidemic of HIV* infection and disease is having an increasingly far-reaching effect on the lives of women here in the United States and throughout the world. Although HIV has affected women from the very beginning of the epidemic, its initial impact was relatively small and went largely unrecognized. Today's situation is very different. According to the World Health Organization, women now comprise one-third of all cases of AIDS worldwide. Here in the United States, women are the fastest-growing group of new cases of AIDS. The total number of women reported to have AIDS in 1980 was 18. Between September 1988 and August 1989, 3,451 cases among women were reported. During the same period of the following year, another 4,486 cases were reported. As of September 1990, the cumulative number of AIDS cases reported among women reached 13,807. The number of AIDS cases among women increases substantially each year, primarily as a result of transmission through intravenous (IV) drug use and unprotected heterosexual intercourse (mainly with partners who use IV drugs).

As a service provider, your work will inevitably be affected by AIDS, even if it is not at present. Whether your focus is on domestic violence, displaced homemakers, sexual assault, jobs-skills development/training, reproductive health, or some other area of direct service for women, the impact of the epidemic will be felt. Those who provide services in communities where other kinds of health, social, and economic problems exist (which are *most* service providers) will experience the greatest impact, but we will *all* be affected eventually.

According to the World Health Organization, women now comprise one-third of all cases of AIDS worldwide.

---

* HIV, the Human Immunodeficiency Virus, is the virus believed to cause AIDS (Acquired Immune Deficiency Syndrome).

WCAP's goal is to stimulate increased advocacy, coalition-building, and comprehensive support for the thousands of women already impacted by the epidemic.

Whether it's the rape survivor's fear that she may be at risk as a result of the assault, the battered woman whose boyfriend insists on having sex without a condom (also known as "unprotected sex"), the displaced homemaker whose son has just been diagnosed with AIDS, or the co-worker in your agency who is infected with HIV, the effects of this epidemic will continue to take many unforeseen forms and will have an ever-increasing impact on the women you serve. Some of you are already facing these issues in your community, while others still have time to plan a response in advance. As with many issues, once your clients know your program is able to address HIV-related issues effectively and sensitively, you may discover that many of the women you serve are already being affected.

In the spring of 1987, Women's Action Alliance developed a project to support and encourage campus-based and independent multi-service women's centers to become involved in the fight against AIDS. The Women's Centers and AIDS Project (WCAP) arose from the concern that the epidemic was taking an increasingly heavy toll on women and that very few services and prevention programs were being specifically designed with women's needs in mind. It was our conviction that community-based women's centers were ideal places to provide HIV education and services that would be sensitive to and appropriate for women in a variety of communities and settings. As the project developed, we saw that community-based organizations and women's centers *could* play a significant role in working to provide valuable HIV-related services for women and their families.

The primary mission of the Women's Centers and AIDS Project is to help women's centers and other community-based organizations to respond to the increasing demand by women for HIV-related information, support, counseling, and advocacy. In its first year, WCAP targeted over 500 women's centers and related organizations in New York and New Jersey, states where the numbers of women with AIDS are significantly higher than the national average. The project had two main components: 1) a series of regional trainings for service providers, and 2) the development and dissemination of materials and information for use by women's centers and other groups. The training and materials were intended not only to provide information, but to promote action. We hoped to stimulate increased advocacy, coalition-building, creative approaches to prevention, and comprehensive support for the thousands of women already impacted by the epidemic.

The goals and activities of the project have remained the same in the years since, and WCAP has expanded in order to provide training and materials throughout the United States. This guidebook is part of a series of materials developed to assist grass roots organizations in becoming active on this issue.

The information presented here is primarily intended for service providers in organizations that may have had little or no previous experience with HIV-related issues, but which recognize the urgency of acting quickly to educate and support the women they serve. The guide describes why AIDS is an issue that your organization can and should address, how it may affect the women you serve, and how to respond to their needs. Practical suggestions for taking a wide range of actions will help you consider the degree of involvement that is most appropriate for your organization.

Of course, you will have to find the avenues that are best for your agency, and the strategies most appropriate for the communities you serve. This guidebook does not address all the options available to you, but offers some basic tools for addressing the epidemic. Even if you have already initiated AIDS-related activities, we hope to provide you with new ideas and issues to consider. Regardless of your previous level of involvement, we believe that your future efforts can make a major difference to those you serve during this health crisis.

1

AIDS
Is a Women's Issue

In terms of both the nature of its impact and sheer numbers, the HIV/ AIDS epidemic is becoming an increasingly urgent and complex "women's issue." Since its beginnings in 1981, the devastating impact of this disease on women and their families has steadily increased. This chapter provides an overview of the impact of HIV/ AIDS on women in the United States — both in terms of the rapid growth in the numbers of women affected, and the specific ways in which women experience the problem. This information may be useful in helping to educate your co-workers, clients, and supporters as to the importance of addressing women and AIDS issues in your agency and on a community-wide level.

Economically disadvantaged African American and Hispanic women are disproportionately impacted.

The numbers

The statistics presented in the introduction and those that follow help to convey the magnitude of the epidemic's impact on women. Although the numbers of women impacted continue to change, they give you an idea of the scope of the problem, serve as tools which you can use to persuade others that AIDS *is* a women's issue, and can help you mobilize support for your center's efforts to provide HIV education and services for women. Most local or state health departments publish regular regional updates of AIDS statistics which are available to the public. See Appendix A for information about how to obtain the national monthly *HIV/AIDS Surveillance Report*, which is available free of charge from the National AIDS Information Clearinghouse.

According to a 1990 study by the federal Centers for Disease Control, the AIDS death rate among U.S. women between the ages of 15 and 44 quadrupled between 1985 and 1988, and will continue to increase at a rapid rate. In 1991, AIDS is expected to become the fifth leading cause of death among U.S. women of childbearing age; in 1988, it was the eighth. In New York City, the epicenter of the epidemic, AIDS is currently the number one killer of women ages 25 to 34. Since 1987, it has been the leading cause of death among African American women ages 15 to 44 in New York and New Jersey. In New York State, the rise in AIDS among women is occurring so quickly that by the mid-90's it is expected to surpass new cases among gay men, who have been the primary population affected by the epidemic thus far.

Just as it is partly shaped by the experiences of gender and sexuality, HIV disease is a reflection of racial and economic disparities in this country as well. Among whites, the AIDS death rate rose from 0.6 per 100,000 women in 1986 to 1.2 in 1988. Among African American women, the rate rose during this period from 4.4 in 1986 to 10.3. That same year, AIDS was responsible for 11% of deaths among

African American women in the U.S. as compared with 3% of white women between the ages of 25 and 34. Young African American women in this country are dying of AIDS at a rate nine times higher than their white counterparts. Latinas are also disproportionately affected — although African Americans and Hispanics comprise only one-fifth of the total U.S. population, African Americans and Latinas make up 72% of all female AIDS cases.

Because HIV can be transmitted from mother to infant in the womb or during childbirth, the figures above also foreshadow the growing incidence of pediatric AIDS. As with women, the majority of pediatric cases are among African Americans and Hispanics: a total of 82% of all cases as of January 1991. In addition to those babies being born with HIV infection, thousands of others will be uninfected, but will be orphaned when their parents die of HIV disease.

Modes of infection

Why do so many women have AIDS and how did they get infected? The vast majority of cases of AIDS among women in this country are either directly or indirectly related to IV drug use. As illustrated below, 51% of all women with AIDS in the U.S. were infected with HIV through intravenous drug use, and 33% through heterosexual inter-course, mostly with male partners who are (or were) IV drug users. Of the remaining cases of AIDS in women, 9% were the result of blood transfusions and the remaining 7% were of "undetermined" cause (*HIV/AIDS Surveillance*, U.S. Department of Health and Human Services, Centers for Disease Control, January 1991).

Figure #1:   **Female exposure catagories**

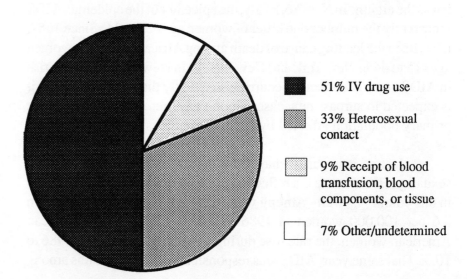

- 51% IV drug use
- 33% Heterosexual contact
- 9% Receipt of blood transfusion, blood components, or tissue
- 7% Other/undetermined

The hidden problem

According to the Centers for Disease Control (CDC), many of the estimated 1.5 million Americans infected with HIV are not aware that they are infected. Many HIV-infected people have no symptoms and have not assessed their risk for past or current exposure to the virus. Still others are aware that they may be at risk, but are afraid to find out for sure by getting the HIV antibody test. They may fear discrimination or feel unable to cope emotionally with what they perceive to be a "death sentence." The fact that so many people are unaware of their HIV status has serious implications for women who are too often advised to protect themselves by merely "knowing" their sexual partner. Asking a partner about his or her sexual or drug-use history may not be very useful if the partner is unaware of — or unwilling to discuss — his or her own possible risk. Many people also believe the dangerous myth that you can tell if someone is infected just by looking at them. Even people who look clean and healthy (and who feel fine) can be infected, and women who do not realize this may unwittingly put themselves at risk by assuming that they can identify "risky" sexual partners on sight. Admonitions to "know" a partner, the assumption that people who are infected are easily identified, and the belief that heterosexuality and marriage are magical protections against HIV/ AIDS sidestep the issues that must be addressed to effectively prevent the spread of HIV: the practice of safer sex, the prevention of IV drug use, and the education of active IV drug users (IVDUs) about the dangers of sharing IV equipment and the risk reduction options available to them.

Because of the long incubation period from the time a person becomes infected with HIV to the onset of symptoms or full-blown AIDS, many people who are infected today will not become sick for many years. That means that even if everyone started using condoms and stopped sharing IV equipment tomorrow, and no new infections occurred in the future, there would *still* be hundreds of thousands of new cases of AIDS over the next two decades, comprised of people who were infected sometime in the past. Unfortunately, we are nowhere near reaching everyone with information, and even farther from the goal of fostering the long-term behavioral changes that will ultimately end or slow the epidemic's spread.

Because only advanced HIV disease, or "AIDS," is reportable in the United States, we can only guess at the numbers of people who are currently infected with HIV and at how many others are ill with less advanced stages of the disease. For every person in the United States who has full-blown AIDS, there are estimated to be 2 to 10 times as many persons whose immune systems have been seriously compromised by the virus, but whose symptoms do not meet the formal case definition for AIDS (this "pre-AIDS" stage of symptomatic infection was formerly known as "ARC," or AIDS-Related Complex). For every person who is immune compromised, there are estimated to be between 2 and 10 persons infected with HIV and asymptomatic. As shown in Figure #2, current AIDS statistics represent only "the tip of the iceberg," and the number of persons who are currently infected and will probably go on to get AIDS is much larger than the total number of current cases of AIDS.

Figure #2:   **AIDS Iceberg**

The AIDS cases counted by the Centers for Disease Control represent only a small portion of the HIV epidemic.

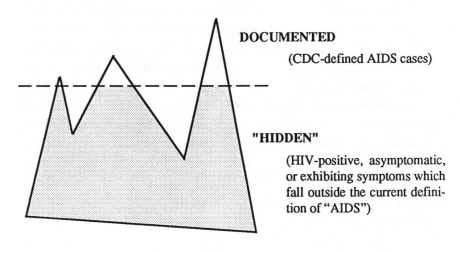

DOCUMENTED

    (CDC-defined AIDS cases)

"HIDDEN"

(HIV-positive, asymptomatic, or exhibiting symptoms which fall outside the current definition of "AIDS")

Undercounting

Many experts believe that, for a variety of reasons, the official statistics significantly underestimate the number of actual AIDS cases in the United States. Understanding the impact of social and economic factors on the reporting of AIDS cases helps us to "read between the lines" of statistical information about this epidemic, and to understand why much still remains hidden. The following are examples of some of the special issues that worsen the problem of undercounting of cases among women:

> ❑ Women are more likely than men to die in the "pre-AIDS" stages of HIV disease. Such cases are not reported as AIDS deaths.
>
> ❑ Case definitions for AIDS were based upon the medical manifestations of male subjects. Some women manifest female-specific HIV-related symptoms such

as vaginal candidiasis, severe pelvic inflammatory disease, abnormal Pap smears, higher rates of and more aggressive forms of cervical cancer, and other gynecological problems related to immune suppression. However, these problems (which also occur among women who are not HIV-positive) are not formally recognized as HIV-related, even in cases where they are. Women are therefore more than twice as likely than men to exhibit HIV-related symptoms that may be misdiagnosed or missed altogether.

❑ Physicians who have not had experience identifying HIV-related illnesses may not always recognize symptoms as being HIV-related. This may be especially true with female clients, because the pervasive myth of "high risk groups" keeps some doctors from perceiving women as "at risk." There are numerous anecdotal cases of women's HIV-related symptoms being attributed to other problems, simply because the physicians did not think to test for HIV, since the woman did not fit the stereotype of a "person with AIDS." Such bias was apparent in the case of a woman in Massachusetts who had tested positive for HIV, but was still told by doctors on numerous occasions that her medical complaints were based on psychological problems, not HIV-related illnesses (*New York Times* 9/23/87, p. A17). (This story, which is only one of many, illustrates the importance of educating health care practitioners about HIV illness in general, and the particular ways it may manifest itself in women. It also highlights the danger of perceiving AIDS as a problem that only affects persons in so-called "high-risk" groups because cases appearing in others may not be recognized. Women with HIV illness risk disease progression when valuable time is lost in diagnosing and treating their condition.)

The problem of failing to recognize HIV-related symptoms may be particularly severe in rural areas where physicians have not yet become practiced in AIDS care, although it is by no means exclusive to these areas.

❑ Private physicians wishing to protect their clients from the stigma associated with this disease may not report AIDS cases as habitually as the health care systems that serve low-income women. This means that AIDS cases among economically privileged persons tend to be undercounted in this country. On the other hand, undercounting also occurs among persons who are totally disenfranchised from the health care system, since they may die before they are even diagnosed. Significant under-reporting of AIDS cases occurs at both ends of the socio-economic spectrum, and is related to the stigma associated with this epidemic, a person's degree of privilege in the society, and the quality of health care they have access to.

Women's isolation is compounded by a social structure in which women are traditionally the providers of care.

AIDS in the lives of women

The epidemic's effect on individual women and their loved ones is devastating: from its damaging effect on physical well-being, to the many psychological, emotional, economic, legal, and social problems it creates and exacerbates. Women are affected in terms of reproductive and civil rights, as caretakers of persons with HIV disease, as concerned parents, as persons with or at risk for HIV infection, and in a variety of other ways. Poverty, lack of access to quality health care, substance abuse, poor housing and nutrition, and lack of power on a societal level and within sexual relationships all create a context in which prevention becomes difficult, and where the impact of the disease itself is compounded. Unlike many gay men, who receive support from the comparatively well-organized and economically privileged gay community, most women with HIV disease experience increased isolation and a lack of organized community support after their diagnosis.

This lack of support is perhaps one of the central differences between the experiences of women and that of many gay men with HIV disease. Women's increased isolation is compounded by a social structure in which women are traditionally the caregivers, and rarely the receivers of care. Women with HIV illness are often so absorbed in caring for a partner or child with AIDS that they put their own health-related needs after those of their loved ones. For many, this can mean not getting the medical care they need until their health has seriously deteriorated. This may be one of the many factors that contribute to women's comparatively brief life expectancy from the time of diagnosis with AIDS — for many, about half that of men. The issues described below also contribute to this striking gap in survival time.

Invisibility of women with HIV

Despite its changing impact on our society, AIDS has been largely portrayed as a gay men's and (male) IV drug users' disease, and its impact on women has been largely obscured. This is a dangerous and misleading myth. A 1989 study by the New York City Department of Health found that more than one-third of the almost 2,000 low-income women interviewed believed that only gay men and IV drug users get AIDS.

The assumption that women are not a significant at-risk population is reflected by:

❑ The lack of gender-specific research and information on the impact of HIV illnesses and the experimental treatments for them on women.

❑ The exclusion of women from some experimental AIDS drug treatment trials and their underrepresentation in others.

❑ The perspective — often promulgated by the mass media and the medical community — that women are vectors of transmission to partners and babies, rather than valued individuals who are themselves at risk of infection and in need of support and care.

❑ The lack of HIV services, outreach efforts, and prevention programs specifically designed to meet women's needs by addressing such issues as caretaking and child care, housing, discrimination, cultural diversity, reproductive and gender-related issues, and poverty.

❑ The underrepresentation of women in media depictions of people with AIDS, or the treatment of women with HIV disease as anomalies or rarities by the mass media.

❑ The lack of preparedness on the part of many direct service organizations to meet the specific needs of HIV-affected women.

❑ The shortage of residential drug treatment programs for women with children.

❑ The lack of childcare and comprehensive family

services throughout the health and AIDS service networks, which prevents many women from availing
themselves of these services.

All of the problems discussed above are compounded in many
regions by seriously overburdened health care systems. Specific
expressions of this problem include severe shortages of bed space,
medical supplies, and care providers in public hospitals, lack of
appropriate insurance coverage for many people in this country, the
absence of nationwide, organized physician and health worker education on HIV in general, the few and limited options that exist for early
preventive medical interventions, as well as the uneven distribution of
medical services that characterizes many rural and urban areas.

The role of community-based organizations

There are several reasons why community groups such as yours are
appropriate and important vehicles for responding to both the larger
context and the individual or community impact of HIV on women by
developing gender-specific prevention, education, and service programs. Grass roots service organizations often serve women who are
at risk for HIV infection or who are experiencing the epidemic through
their families and communities. Many groups work with young,
sexually active women who may be at risk through experimentation
with drugs or sex. Others serve women whose communities are disproportionately affected by the epidemic. And many CBOs are located
in areas where there is a high or growing concentration of AIDS cases
among women. Even if your agency is not serving any of these
populations or working in one of these regions, your clients — and staff
— need to know about an epidemic that is transcending lines of age,
geography, race, class, gender, and sexual identity. Like domestic
violence and rape, the true impact of HIV upon women will remain
hidden until cultural norms change and women feel able to speak about
their experiences more openly. Women's centers and other CBOs that
confront HIV directly can both raise the community's level of awareness and help to identify and support clients who are personally
affected.

Women come to your organization because unlike many
traditional social service agencies, you provide easily accessed, non-
judgmental, empathetic assistance. Perhaps you offer battered women's
programs, rape crisis counseling, job training, parenting support,
health promotion and education, information/referral, or support groups.
HIV education can be effectively integrated into all of these programs.
Like other community-based organizations, women's centers are

trusted service providers, and thus can develop appropriate information and support on HIV in ways that will be acceptable to the communities served. For these reasons, women's centers and other community-based organizations can help insure that women receive the information, support, and services they need to cope with the growing impact of the epidemic.

Most importantly, you have the capacity to reach people who would never walk into an AIDS organization for fear of being stigmatized. By integrating HIV issues into other areas of concern to women, the stigma associated with AIDS can be reduced and the information can reach a much broader audience. That's why the involvement of all kinds of service organizations is so crucial.

The direct services your center provides are probably more than enough to keep it overextended, understaffed, and underfunded. In fact, you may be saying to yourself, "AIDS is an important issue, but there's no way my center can take on one more responsibility right now." Regardless of whether you choose to become involved, one thing you *can* be sure of is that the HIV epidemic will eventually have an impact on your program and your clients in some way. By becoming active now — even to a modest degree — you can help your organization, your staff, and your clients to face the problem. That means creating sensible, caring policies and activities, rather than just responding to crises as they arise. A proactive position may mean working out your confidentiality or discrimination-related policies *before* the need emerges. It might involve increasing the visibility of HIV issues so that the women in your center will feel able to seek your support if they need it. Ideally, it will mean creating a safe and empowering environment both for those who are already impacted by HIV/AIDS as well as those who are not.

The next chapter describes the different opportunities for action in both heavily impacted areas and those where the epidemic seems very far away. It suggests how to determine the service and prevention gaps in your area and how to match them against your clients' needs to develop programs that are right for your constituency *and* your organization. To help you start at a degree of involvement that is appropriate for your agency, it is followed by a listing of over forty HIV-related activities organized into three levels, from very basic to more advanced. We encourage you to test them out and to invent your own.

Women's centers can develop appropriate information and support on HIV in ways that will be acceptable to the communities served.

2

How Women's Centers Can Help

Low incidence regions: opportunities for action

Thus far, the HIV epidemic has hit hardest in America's large cities. Those of you who live and work in rural or suburban regions or smaller cities may feel that since HIV is not a crisis in your area, it's not worth your while to become involved. Why raise issues that don't currently exist — especially when there are so many other pressing problems to deal with? The answer is that because this epidemic does not respect county lines, chances are that you have *already* dealt with women who have been directly impacted in some way by HIV, even if you don't know it and they haven't talked about it. If you live in an area where few people have been affected, you are lucky; unfortunately, the likelihood is that this will change. Over the coming years, the epidemic is expected to continue in currently impacted areas, while dramatically affecting regions that are not, at present, considered "high incidence."

Between 1988 and 1989, the federal Centers for Disease Control reported a 35.4% increase in the number of reported AIDS cases in cities with fewer than 100,000 persons, as compared with a 4.6% growth rate for metropolitan areas of 1 million people or more. In other words, AIDS is now increasing at a much faster rate in rural communities than in large urban centers, although the total numbers in rural areas are, in most cases, still much smaller. A National AIDS Commission report released in August 1990 found that in Georgia, for example, the number of women with AIDS in rural areas is almost as high as it is in Atlanta. The "explosion" of HIV disease in rural areas is exacerbated by increased levels of discrimination (resulting in large part from a lack of AIDS education), the lack of awareness on the part of health care providers about existing AIDS treatments, and the precarious positions of rural hospitals and other health-related facilities in such regions.

The best way to keep your area's caseload low is to implement energetic prevention efforts *now*. Another reason for doing general community education in areas with few cases of HIV/AIDS is that when such cases do arise — and they inevitably will — your community can respond intelligently, rather than out of ignorance and fear. Getting to your community before the epidemic does (or early on) will save lives and lay the groundwork for appropriate, compassionate responses to the local problems brought about or compounded by the epidemic.

Service providers in heavily affected areas often remark upon how rapidly and dramatically the epidemic seemed to develop in those areas, allowing little time for the planning and implementation of appropriate support services and programs. Those of you working in

Chances are you have *already* dealt with women who have been impacted by AIDS, even if you don't know it.

low-incidence areas are fortunate enough to have an opportunity to assess your community's needs and organize locally for strong prevention efforts, appropriate HIV/AIDS policies, and comprehensive service delivery, *in advance*. Groups like yours can have an impact by:

> ❑ Making HIV prevention a high-profile topic in your region;
>
> ❑ vigorously educating the community about HIV discrimination;
>
> ❑ developing special programs and materials in conjunction with your community;
>
> ❑ integrating HIV-related information and services into your program's other activities;
>
> ❑ organizing local or regional work groups to plan strategies to overcome obstacles to reducing high-risk behavior;
>
> ❑ organizing educational activities for local health and social service providers, schools, hospitals, and other agencies that serve the public;
>
> ❑ networking with other community leaders and organizations to encourage their support of appropriate HIV-related services and activities; and
>
> ❑ working in your community to make safer sex and the prevention and treatment of drug abuse the norm.

While you are in a good position to make a difference, you may face the challenge of convincing your community leaders and constituency that this problem should be addressed now. Providing examples of how rapidly the numbers are increasing in other rural regions or small cities might be one way to help break through resistance. The key lies in helping people understand that facing HIV now may prevent much loss of life and anguish later. You have the opportunity to learn from what has happened elsewhere, and to develop creative approaches that are specially tailored to suit your community.

Heavily impacted regions: opportunities for action

In areas where large numbers of people have been affected, there are challenges as well as opportunities for the women's center or CBO interested in offering HIV-related activities. Most high-incidence regions already have active AIDS organizations and other community groups which can be important sources of information, technical assistance, and guidance to you as you begin to work in this area. However, even in communities where many active organizations exist, there are sure to be many unmet needs. There is more than enough work to go around, but it's important to find out what needs *are* being met in order to avoid duplicating services.

You can start by contacting other AIDS organizations in your area as well as community-based organizations who may be doing AIDS work along with their other activities. Appendices A and B include listings of New York, New Jersey, and national AIDS organization(s). Your local health department, American Red Cross, hospital, and/or AIDS task force can probably lead you to other groups doing relevant work in your area. Making these contacts allows you to find out what needs remain unmet in the community, and puts you in touch with resources that may be supportive of your efforts.

Networking *before* creating programs helps establish a cooperative relationship between groups. One way to cultivate this cooperation is to meet periodically with other local CBOs and AIDS service organizations to share information, coordinate services, and form a strong base for doing local advocacy for funding and resources. Such coalitions may already exist in your community. If you are helping to form a new coalition, invite persons with relevant experience to share, even if their expertise is not AIDS-specific: those who have been active in the women's and minority health movements, community organizing, drug prevention and drug treatment programs, health education, and related activities can enrich your efforts by offering diverse skills and broadened perspectives on the issues.

Determining the needs and interests of the women you serve

Before planning HIV-related programs for the women who come to your center or for your community-at-large, it is important to understand the needs of those who are currently using your services. Often, eliciting community participation at the outset avoids the creation of inappropriate programs. A combined knowledge of your community's needs and of the HIV services in your area allows you to develop relevant programs without duplicating existing activities and services.

**Start by having
all center staff
attend some edu-
cational forums
or training on
HIV.**

The first step is to find out what your clients need and want. A "client needs assessment survey" will probably make you aware of a greater demand for programs and services than you can meet. Remember that while you cannot respond to everyone's needs, you can begin to meet some. Even sponsoring a series of meetings or organizing one support group can help increase the visibility and lessen the stigma of HIV in your community while meeting real demands. Gathering information about your community's concerns is important, since it allows your program to work with others to develop or advocate for new programs or policies that will address these needs.

If your organization wants to plan some small events or activities, you may not need to survey your clients first. However, by encouraging women to personalize the HIV issue, a survey can raise awareness just by posing questions. If you do plan to hand out a survey, be prepared for HIV-related questions and concerns, both from the women you serve and from your staff. We suggest you start by having *all* of your staff, paid and unpaid, attend some educational forums or training on HIV. Start with basic information (sometimes known as "AIDS 101"). It may also be advisable to cover special issues such as organizational and administrative policies, counseling, HIV antibody testing, medical issues, bereavement, discrimination, and legal concerns. The level and type of training needed by your staff will depend on how involved your organization decides to become. Local AIDS programs and health departments can often provide such training, or will refer you to appropriate agencies.

Many readers are well versed in conducting assessments of their community's needs. The following discussion of how to conduct a client needs assessment is included for those who have not had previous experience in this area.

A sample client needs assessment that can be modified for your organization is included in Appendix C. It can answer such questions as: Do the women you serve need basic HIV and health information? Do they want to learn how to teach their children about AIDS? Are they interested in a safer sex support group? Are they seeking other types of information and support?

Tailor the questions to the local situation and create questions that make sense for *your* clients. For example, if you work with displaced homemakers, include questions that are specific to them, such as how to talk with their children and how to deal with safer sex and dating, or concerns related to HIV in the workplace. Focus group discussions may be useful in figuring out how best to design the questionnaire, what to ask, and how to ask it.

In order to increase the participation of the women you serve:

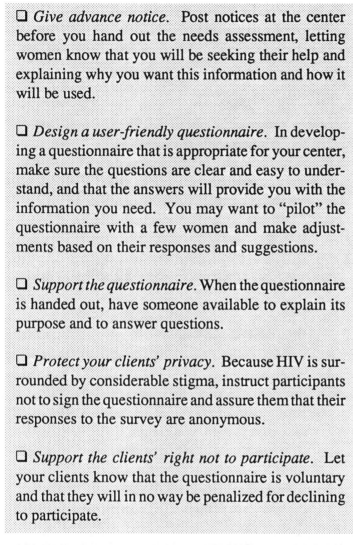

❑ *Give advance notice.* Post notices at the center before you hand out the needs assessment, letting women know that you will be seeking their help and explaining why you want this information and how it will be used.

❑ *Design a user-friendly questionnaire.* In developing a questionnaire that is appropriate for your center, make sure the questions are clear and easy to understand, and that the answers will provide you with the information you need. You may want to "pilot" the questionnaire with a few women and make adjustments based on their responses and suggestions.

❑ *Support the questionnaire.* When the questionnaire is handed out, have someone available to explain its purpose and to answer questions.

❑ *Protect your clients' privacy.* Because HIV is surrounded by considerable stigma, instruct participants not to sign the questionnaire and assure them that their responses to the survey are anonymous.

❑ *Support the clients' right not to participate.* Let your clients know that the questionnaire is voluntary and that they will in no way be penalized for declining to participate.

You can hand out these questionnaires along with other intake materials when women first come to your center, and have the questionnaire deposited in a separate "response box" in a common area. Or you can simply leave a pile of surveys on a table in the waiting room and ask incoming clients to fill one out and return it the next time they come to the center. You can also encourage center staff to distribute them at workshops and events.

After collecting the questionnaires, match the concerns presented against what already exists in the community. If the needs expressed are not being met elsewhere, how can you best meet them? If they *are* already being addressed in your area, how can you publicize their availability to your clients and help to increase their accessibility to the women you serve?

Shortly after considering these questions, create some kind of

Your timely response enriches the bond between your organization and the community it serves.

follow-up activity or event in response to the assessments. For example, if some women expressed concern about talking to their children about HIV, you might sponsor a workshop which would include basic HIV information, special issues for children, tips on how to talk to young people about AIDS, and an opportunity for participants to do role playing in which they can practice having conversations with their children. A workshop like this will not only address a specific issue presented by the women you serve, but will provide a forum for women to meet others who share their concern. Your timely response shows your clients that their comments were taken seriously and encourages their participation in future activities. It enriches the bond between your organization and the community it serves by demonstrating that the services you deliver are responsive to the needs expressed by the women who utilize them.

Determining whether women's needs are being met in your community

Once you know what kind of services or information the women in your community would like to have, it's helpful to get a profile of the services that exist in your area. Before referring women to other programs, it's important to know that your clients would be welcome, that their needs would be met, and that the services offered are appropriate for them. For example, you should know whether your local AIDS service programs make childcare available. Does it have female counselors? Do they speak the languages spoken by the women in your community? Is the staff sensitized to the special ways that HIV affects women? A community needs assessment like the one in Appendix D helps clarify whether such services exist. Getting the answers to questions like these will help you identify areas of need and become an informed advocate for women's concerns in the community.

Once you have collected this information, it may be used in any or all of the following ways:

❑ To strengthen the quality of your information and referral resources;

❑ to publicize existing services for women among your clients and in the community;

❑ to identify gaps in services for women and to use this documentation as a program-planning, fund-raising, grant-writing, or advocacy tool;

❏ to work with existing groups to improve the accessibility and appropriateness of local services for women; and

❏ to decide which unmet needs your center might best address.

As with the first questionnaire, the community needs assessment survey is intended as a point of departure for you to create your own form. This second questionnaire is much more involved than the one for clients. A broad range of issues needs to be considered in order to do a thorough analysis of the services in your area. You may not be able to do such a lengthy survey, but you *can* zero in on specific issues by asking only those questions which might help you sharpen the quality of your referrals. Likewise, you can specify questions that involve services your center might be able to provide. For example, if you are thinking about initiating a women's support group, start by investigating whether anyone else in your region runs one, and what kind of group it is. While there may already be a support group for women with AIDS, there may not be anything for women who are HIV-positive, or for female friends, caretakers, or partners of people with HIV disease. You could also find out if any transportation or childcare needs remain unmet for the women in your area who use these services, and then try to fill those gaps.

There are at least two ways to implement the community needs assessment. You can telephone key persons at local AIDS and other community-based organizations and ask them the relevant questions listed on the survey. Or you can set up meetings with these service providers and work through the questionnaire together, deciding as a group where the gaps are, and planning a coordinated response. Setting up work groups cultivates rapport and can help groups move together on important issues by reducing competition and fostering a cooperative effort on local HIV prevention and service provision.

Note: Certain annotated AIDS service directories provide some of the information that the sample questionnaire in Appendix D is designed to obtain, so find out what local listings exist before undertaking your research. Be aware, however, that few directories are focused specifically on women's needs, so you'll probably still need to do some follow-up to ascertain if the programs listed are appropriate for the women you serve. Gather as much information as you can from existing sources and then supplement the information with your phone survey or work group approach.

3

Activities

This chapter provides examples of different HIV-related activities that your center can offer to the women it serves. Included are three levels of activity:

❑ The first level focuses on increasing basic AIDS awareness among the staff and clients of your organization. It means establishing your agency as a "safe" place to talk about HIV. Activities on this level require a relatively small amount of staff time and fiscal expense.

❑ The second level of activity integrates HIV education and services into the programs you already provide. Whether your programs involve job training, parenting support, or reproductive health care, these activities suggest how to connect HIV to the other important issues that you address.

❑ The third level involves creating special programs and activities on HIV that stand apart from other programs in your organization. Targeted, HIV-specific programs enable you to highlight HIV as a topic of urgent importance and to mobilize special resources toward prevention, education, and support.

This list of activities is meant to provide you with hints on how to get started, not to offer step-by-step guidelines on implementation. Since you are already knowledgeable about how to carry out different kinds of programs at your center, this guide offers some of the specific HIV-related issues to be aware of before you start.

By beginning to address the health crisis at your center, you are likely to raise unforeseen issues and questions among both clients and staff. Therefore, it is important to begin by training your staff on basic HIV information as well as sexual and drug-related issues, since understanding these is integral to understanding the epidemic. Staff training should also include information about HIV antibody testing, a review of community resources, values clarification about controversial issues, and skills development in talking with clients about such topics. It is also important to be sensitive to the staff's feelings and fears about dealing with these complex issues. By offering accurate information and a chance to express their concerns, you will provide them with the tools and confidence to deal appropriately with the women they serve. Such training can usually be provided by your local AIDS task force, health department, drug prevention group, or family planning organization.

Basic information and referral resources should be available to women who want to know more.

Some organizations may want to designate at least one staff member (or community volunteer) to coordinate HIV-related activities. This person may take on the responsibility for gathering information and becoming knowledgeable about the issue, organizing staff trainings, networking with local AIDS organizations and other community-based groups, and orchestrating your agency's activities in this area.

It is also a good idea to have some basic information and referral resources available as a backup for women who want more information or who need to be referred to an HIV service provider. Contact your local AIDS hotline or department of health for information about services available in your area. Appendix A contains selections from WCAP's annotated *Guide to AIDS Education Materials*, which lists books, posters, videos, pamphlets, and other relevant materials for women. This listing will help you locate some of the materials mentioned below.

Level I: Increase HIV awareness in your program

Without spending a great deal of time and energy, you can send a message to your community that it's all right to talk about HIV in your organization, and that you want to be supportive of women who are being affected by the epidemic. Below are some actions your can take toward this end.

❑ Display educational posters to indicate the center's commitment to the HIV issue and to help increase the overall awareness and visibility of the subject. Most AIDS organizations and state or local health departments distribute posters;

❑ Show HIV education videos in waiting rooms, lounges, drop-in centers, etc. Videos are available at low cost or free of charge from some AIDS service agencies and health departments. These organizations — and some video distributors — will also loan videos temporarily to community groups who lack the resources to purchase them. It can be helpful to have a speaker available to answer questions and to "process" people's feelings after a video is shown;

❑ Distribute free brochures and booklets on various topics at a visible and accessible location in your organization. Printed materials on HIV are available in a variety of languages, reading levels, and designs, and cover a wide range of topics and issues;

❏ Keep an ongoing file or "library" containing books, newspaper articles, videos, and information on women and HIV (or HIV generally) for use by clients and staff. Publicize the library and related activities within the community. Involve the community by requesting that people donate articles and information of interest. This not only insures that the library has information from a variety of sources, but encourages community participation in its success. It also keeps people on the lookout for AIDS information, which makes the topic a visible one. You can further stimulate interest by planning discussions and educational forums on recent HIV-related news and events;

❏ Distribute free condoms, water-based lubricants, dental dams, and safer sex brochures at an accessible location — some organizations keep a goldfish bowl filled in their waiting area or common space. Have someone available to explain how to use the prevention materials you are providing. Make sure this person is trained to discuss safer sex issues in a non-judgmental and relaxed manner which encourages questions and open discussion. (For more information about condoms and dental dams, see the section on "Negotiating for information and safer sex" in the next chapter);

❏ Include HIV information and announcements of related programs in each issue of your center's newsletter. If the newsletter is theme-oriented, publish an entire issue on women and AIDS. Solicit contributions from local HIV educators and the staff of your program, as well as asking the women you serve to write about their own thoughts, feelings, and concerns. Include a "Commonly Asked Questions" section or a special resource list for women in your area, along with the local AIDS hotline's phone number;

❏ Set up an "AIDS Alert" chart to keep the women you serve informed about what is happening with HIV/AIDS in your area. The chart can include local information and statistics from your state's department of health. If your area's cases are high in number, the chart will serve to reinforce local concern about the issue. If numbers are low, try to obtain AIDS statistics for other areas similar to your own. Include information on related issues such as IV drug use, teen pregnancy, and sexually-transmitted diseases (STDs). This kind of information helps people (especially those who do not live in HIV epicenters) to see that HIV affects their community, too;

❏ On campus, set up an HIV information booth or table in a

Include HIV prevention information in each issue of your center's newsletter.

Integrate HIV information and education into existing support groups.

heavily trafficked area. Make prevention literature, condoms, and referral information available at the booth, and staff it with someone who is able to answer questions;

❑ Invite a panel of women who are directly impacted by HIV to speak to your organization;

❑ Information tables work in other settings, too — from supermarkets and subway entrances to shopping malls and school meetings;

❑ Ask campus and community bookstores to display HIV prevention posters and to carry books and other materials;

❑ If you have meeting space to spare, offer to donate it to a local HIV-related group for weekly meetings or special events.

Level II: Integrate HIV education and services into pre-existing programs

One of the main benefits of integrating HIV education into programs that already exist is that you can reach women who would not normally attend an AIDS-focused event. By taking a "holistic" approach to HIV prevention — placing it within the context of empowerment, support, and skills-building — the issue is more likely to be seen as relevant and interconnected to the other concerns women face. With the assistance of local HIV educators and programs, you can:

❑ Offer your agency's service providers and support group leaders training, information, materials, and technical assistance on introducing HIV information into counseling, group discussions, and other ongoing services and programs;

❑ Train leaders of self-help groups for battered women and others to include advocacy for safer sex along with other empowerment issues. Your local AIDS service organization or health department may be able to offer training free of charge;

❑ Integrate HIV information and education into pre-existing support groups by means of discussions that focus on the relationship between HIV and the support group's theme (e.g. single mothers, domestic violence, drug prevention, sexuality, parenting, etc.);

❑ Establish an HIV component in the center's ongoing information and referral service, including sources of educational print materials, films, and information about local service, treatment, and support programs;

❑ Infuse HIV information into literacy, English as a Second Language (ESL), job training, and General Equivalency Diploma (GED) classes by using reading, writing, and typing materials and exercises that focus on HIV, drugs, and sexuality. You can use pre-existing HIV prevention materials or amend these materials to suit the specific needs of your population;

❑ Integrate prevention information and "consciousness raising" about HIV-related pregnancy issues into other activities at family planning clinics, teen pregnancy and new mothers programs, presentations on reproductive issues, and other relevant programs;

❑ If adolescents are served, provide special programs on HIV for teenagers, including rap and arts groups, peer counseling programs, and videos made by and for young audiences;

❑ Distribute HIV education materials along with your own organization's fliers when you do outreach at local block parties, country fairs, and community events;

❑ If your program offers services where special HIV-related concerns might arise (such as sexual assault counseling), develop a brochure for clients which addresses the relationship between these issues;

❑ Make HIV information available to individuals who might not attend a meeting exclusively focused on AIDS by incorporating the information into general events, discussions, and fairs on health, mental health, stress reduction, nutrition, substance abuse, parenting, and related issues;

❑ Set up a general, ongoing support group for women in which a forum is created for them to talk about the immediate issues that they are dealing with in their lives that are not necessarily AIDS-related. While addressing other themes, try to also integrate HIV information and prevention skills in the context of assertiveness, communication, negotiation skills, health, or sexuality-related issues;

❑ Through campus-based women's centers and other student programs, HIV education can be integrated into other class-

At campus-based women's centers, HIV education can be integrated into other classroom activities.

room activities. For example, at San Francisco State University, student writers and photographers worked on a semester-long project to create a collection of photographs and essays on people who care for people with AIDS. Group activities such as this can be useful for sensitizing students to the impact of the epidemic and driving home the importance of prevention and education;

❑ Include HIV/AIDS as a topic if you sponsor monthly information meetings, a brown-bag lunch series, or some other regular group event.

Level III: Implement special HIV activities

If your organization has the financial resources and personnel to develop specific, "free standing" HIV education, prevention, or support programs, it can:

❑ Establish an advisory committee of local HIV service providers and advocates for women's issues to advise and provide support for your organization's activities;

❑ Establish a local task force of people who work in HIV-related jobs, which can meet periodically to provide up-to-date information on an issue of interest and promote networking, resource-sharing, and support opportunities for participants;

❑ Create a community HIV task force comprised of women who use the center and program staff to design activities, establish priorities, recommend policy, and advocate for the needs of women;

❑ Focus forums and guided discussion on such topics as "Basic HIV/AIDS Information," "How Is AIDS a Women's Issue?", "Talking with our Partners about AIDS," "African American Women and HIV," "Drugs and HIV," "Preventing Drug Abuse and AIDS in our Community," "Talking with our Children about AIDS," "Talking with our Children about Death and Dying," "Talking with Other Parents about AIDS," "Dating During an Epidemic," "Questions and Concerns," "Lesbians and HIV," "Issues for Caregivers," "AIDS in Rural Areas," etc.;

❑ Offer ongoing individual counseling, support groups or workshops on negotiating with a sexual partner. Role play and discussion topics might include: becoming empowered to talk about sensitive issues; coping with a substance-abusing partner; the meaning of trust; when and how to ask difficult questions; how to deal with the answers received; how to make healthy decisions using the information available; how to stick with a decision; and eroticizing safer sex;

❑ Set up "buddy,"* transportation, childcare, meal delivery, or care partner services for women with HIV disease;

❑ Conduct ongoing individual counseling and/or discussion groups on safer sex, focusing on: safer-sex techniques; cultural issues; building negotiation skills; becoming empowered to advocate for one's health and well being; dealing with a partner's resistance; feelings about safer sex and changing sexual behavior; planning ahead for safer sex; the barriers for practicing birth control in general, and to using condoms in particular; the barriers women face in trying to take an equal role in sexual decision-making, etc.;

❑ Offer special support groups for women with HIV illness and/or who are HIV-positive;

❑ Offer support groups for women who are caregivers to people with HIV disease;

❑ Offer ongoing or short-term programs on death, dying, and bereavement;

❑ Invite speakers on such topics as the impact of HIV on the local community; the effect of alcohol and other mood-altering substances on high-risk behaviors; the effect of HIV on the lesbian community; HIV and reproductive rights; HIV-related discrimination; HIV, children, and the schools; and other topics as requested by attendees;

❑ Offer discussion groups on "To test or not to test";

❑ Offer a public forum entitled, "Everything You Always Wanted to Know about AIDS. . . But Were Afraid to Ask" in which audience members write down questions anonymously and pass them up to an AIDS educator who will read and discuss each one with the group;

---

* "Buddies" are trained volunteers who provide companionship and practical assistance (such as shopping, cleaning, or transportation to and from medical appointments) to people with HIV disease.

What information do we want other women to have? How can we convey that information in a way that will be understood and accepted? How would *we* want to receive such information?

❑ Do role plays with clients — teens or adults — to practice asking their partners to use condoms, telling them they are HIV-positive, speaking with doctors, applying for insurance, or talking to their children about HIV. If the role-playing model is successful, take it "on the road" to perform for other women's groups in your organization or to the community;

❑ To increase audience involvement, try "stop action" role plays. "Freeze" the role play in the middle and ask audience members to discuss what they think will happen next. In addition to increasing the audience's involvement with the role play and the issues it addresses, the "stop action" format provides a forum for participants to "brainstorm," share ideas on how to approach different situations, and actively consider the implications of these issues in their own lives;

❑ Another variation of the role play is to do "round robin," where after a few minutes a different person takes on each role, providing participants with an opportunity to observe several styles and approaches to handling a specific issue. This approach also gives the facilitator and group more material to discuss and allows more women to become actively involved;

❑ Encourage members of the women's center to create their own educational materials by designing posters, literature, and other materials. A workshop on this topic could address the following questions: What information do we want other women to have? How can we convey that information in a way that will be understood and accepted? How would *we* want to receive such information? A project of this kind draws on a variety of skills, reinforces participants' knowledge of the issues, and helps them think about what works in creating useful materials. The final product can then be used to increase visibility of and knowledge of the issue among their peers. This activity can be made into a contest with a prize (First prize: an assortment of multicolored and other "fun" condoms and safer sex supplies!);

❑ Sponsor poster, pamphlet or "rap music" contests with an HIV theme in high schools, prisons, drug treatment programs, or other settings in the community;

❑ If your program works with children, provide them with age-appropriate basic HIV education, and follow up by sponsoring a contest where they design simple posters on various aspects of HIV (e.g. why you shouldn't discriminate against people with HIV, how to prevent the spread of HIV, why you don't need to be afraid of people with HIV, etc.);

❑ If your agency has outdoor space, offer to have an HIV education or drug prevention mural put up in that spot. You can have a local graffiti artist do the job — or better still, work with your clients or their children in developing, designing, and painting the piece;

❑ Train members of staff and/or at-risk clients to do trainings themselves. Teach women who come to the center to do HIV education and outreach in their communities. Many HIV/AIDS organizations provide such training;

❑ Set up an outreach program where women from the center run small workshops or meetings in homes, laundromats, social clubs, church groups, beauty parlors, shopping centers, and other places where women can be reached. Throughout the country, a model based on the "Tupperware Party" is being used in women's homes, where a comfortable, non-threatening atmosphere supports open discussion about sexual issues, HIV prevention techniques, and other health concerns;

❑ On campus, conduct outreach to sororities, fraternities, and dormitories. Ask sororities to sponsor safer sex education parties, video showings, AIDS fund-raisers, or other activities that raise the issue of HIV prevention on campus. Visit dorms to hand out safer sex materials and answer questions in an informal setting;

❑ Remember that college campuses and schools are also good places to target substance abuse prevention activities — and to highlight the connections between HIV disease and drug and alcohol abuse;

❑ Contact local media (i.e. radio, TV, newspapers, newsletters) to publicize your efforts in any of the above areas. This helps you reach people who might not otherwise know about your center or its programs, and creates a wider forum for communicating information on women and HIV disease;

❑ Create a "Women's Media Watch Committee" to encourage your local media to feature stories about how the epidemic affects women and to monitor their coverage of HIV-related issues generally. Organize letter-writing or telephone campaigns either to support constructive coverage or criticize irresponsible or counterproductive reporting (such as journalism which scapegoats women or prostitutes). Because the

Make your local media accountable for the type of HIV-related reporting they do.

media impacts so heavily on public opinion, it will benefit the women you serve to make your local media accountable for the type of HIV-related reporting they do;

❑ Co-sponsor support efforts for men interested in practicing and maintaining safer sex in their relationships with women. Teaching heterosexual women about safer sex and helping them build negotiation skills will only go so far. Their male partners must also be given support and encouragement to change their sexual behavior. If your center is not an appropriate place to facilitate targeted prevention efforts for men, explore the possibility of co-sponsoring such an event with another local group, such as the local pool hall, social club, bowling alley, gym, or YMCA;

❑ Organize oral history or other creative documentation projects for HIV-positive women and women with AIDS;

❑ Provide supportive activities for the children of women who have HIV disease;

❑ Establish an "Adopt-a-Caregiver" program utilizing a less intensive form of the "buddy" model to provide support to caregivers;

❑ Create a respite program for caregivers, utilizing volunteers who can spend a few hours with persons with HIV disease so that the primary caregivers can have some time for themselves.

The preceding suggestions highlight some of the many directions your organization can take or may already have taken in trying to make HIV/AIDS a more visible, better understood issue. There are as many ways to convey HIV information as there are people who need to receive it, so be creative and design your own outreach formats. *The Women's Centers and AIDS Project is always interested in sharing new outreach ideas, so if you come up with something you'd like to share with other women's groups, please write to us at the project.*

4

AIDS Is Not
the Same for Everyone:
Fostering a
Community-Based Response

Although AIDS has become a highly visible subject, there remains a striking lack of awareness of its impact on women and various cultural communities. The dominant approach has been to target prevention information to a "general population," assumed to be uniform in cultural background, social mores, and life experience. This type of approach means that prevention efforts, such as pamphlets, television advertisements, and bus posters, are often irrelevant to the experience of women, people of color, and the economically disadvantaged. The success of HIV prevention campaigns specially designed by and for the gay male community exemplifies the value of targeting information to specific groups; it also highlights the importance of communities *developing their own strategies for education and prevention.* Health maintenance and HIV prevention are empowerment issues involving community-based creation of prevention messages and approaches for responding to this epidemic. As a service provider, you can supply HIV-related information and resources so that the community you serve can develop its own materials and strategies.

By understanding some of the specific ways that HIV impacts on women, and how it has traditionally been addressed in many mainstream HIV education efforts, you can better identify the right fit between the community's needs and whatever efforts you may choose to undertake. This understanding will also help you to select or create HIV education materials that are targeted to the community you serve, or to adapt existing materials. The following issues are commonly used by AIDS educators as examples of why the so-called "general audience" approach to HIV prevention fails to address the diverse needs of women, and thus limits the effectiveness of these campaigns. The outline also indicates some of the wider problems with the ways our society has "constructed" or thought about HIV/AIDS thus far.

Pamphlets, television advertisements, and bus posters, often fail to speak to the experience of women, people of color, and the economically disadvantaged.

The myth of risk groups

Some HIV prevention materials continue to reflect the myth that only people in "high-risk groups" (e.g. gay men, prostitutes, IV drug users, etc.) are vulnerable to AIDS. In fact, one's identity has nothing to do with getting AIDS: *behavior* is the sole determinant of risk. Gay men, for instance, are not inherently at risk, just as women are not automatically free of it. A prostitute who routinely practices safer sex will be at lower risk than a married woman who has unprotected sex with her HIV-infected husband. In other words, risk is based entirely on behavior, as opposed to who someone is or how she identifies herself. The risk group myth is dangerous to everyone, but it has proven especially dangerous to women, many of whom feel immune just by virtue of their gender, race, socio-economic status, religious standing, or marital status. Emphasizing risk factors and risk behaviors and moving away from misleading phrases like "risk groups" can help empower women to take control of their lives and health.

A false sense of "us" and "them" leads to discriminatory prevention policies.

One of the secondary dangers of the "risk group" concept is the notion that only certain "types" of people should be concerned with HIV prevention, thus encouraging a false sense of "us" and "them" that often leads to counterproductive and discriminatory prevention policies. The belief that only "certain" people need to practice safer sex leads to the stigmatization of those who try to incorporate this behavior into their daily lives, thereby making it difficult for people to protect themselves. A more effective approach is to work toward making safer sex the norm, as it has become in many parts of the gay male community. This means women encouraging one another to advocate for safer sex with their partners, and men being supported and encouraged to use condoms — making safer sex and condom use the expected behaviors, and empowering women to reject sexual partners who insist on putting their partners (and themselves) at risk. Service providers can support their community's efforts to foster new norms for positive health behaviors by working within the existing cultural frameworks and belief systems of that community.

Culture and language appropriateness

Women of color have been disproportionately affected by the HIV epidemic, and its dramatic toll on African American and Latino communities continues to rise. Though less information is available about AIDS in Native American and Asian American communities, we do know that the number of cases in those communities continues to grow. Asian Americans and Native Americans share the burden of cultural bias, poverty, and discrimination with African American and Latino communities, while also suffering from a lack of visibility *within* communities of color.

Offering a diversity of materials (e.g., different reading levels, different languages, information presented in different styles and reflecting a variety of value systems) is an important part of making sure HIV education reaches everyone. Prevention materials aimed at a specific group should utilize the cultural cues of that group, stressing prevention within the context of that group's value system and emphasizing cultural strengths which can be marshalled toward protecting the group from HIV disease. This may include visual cues, cultural idioms, and recognizable symbols, the invocation of cultural pride, and appropriate use of language. To help you meet your community's needs, the Women's Center and AIDS Project has produced a resource list of free or low-cost pamphlets, books, posters, and videotapes that are geared to women and people of color. This annotated list includes materials designed for women in different cultural groups, as well as adolescents, college-age women, lesbians, and other populations. Themes addressed include AIDS in the workplace, legal/discrimination issues, treatment and self-care for people with HIV disease, the HIV antibody test, prison issues, and many more. If you want to make materials like these available at your center, information on how to order the list is located in Appendix A, which includes an updated and abbreviated version of the 14-page resource list.

Going beyond pamphlets and posters

Providing written and visual educational materials can be a good way to introduce HIV information to the women you serve. However, no brochure can address all women's needs and questions, support women in changing their behavior, or deal with the many psychosocial issues raised by the epidemic. Since many women have by now been reached by some of the "general audience" HIV education campaigns (through the former Surgeon General's mass mailing, television, and other media), our goal must be to help women *use* this information to protect themselves and others. Educational materials are best used as complements to other types of HIV prevention activities, such as individual or group support, workshops, and other interactive, dynamic projects such as those described in the previous chapter.

Integrating AIDS prevention efforts

In order for HIV information to have real meaning, it should be integrated into other areas of concern in women's lives. For instance, if some women attend a single mothers' support group at your organization, HIV is not likely to be the group's main area of concern, but it can be made relevant by discussing prevention as it relates to dating issues and safer sex, educating one's child about sexuality, deciding whether to have another child, and other childrearing and parenthood issues. Many women will not attend an "AIDS workshop" because they do not see themselves as being at risk or because of their fear of being stigmatized. However, a workshop on "Parenting Skills," "Women and Health," or "Surviving the '90's," where HIV and other important information can be integrated into a larger and less overwhelming topic, will provide women with the information and support they need. Integrating HIV education into other kinds of activities also gives women the chance to apply HIV-related concerns to their daily lives, rather than perceiving them as distant issues unconnected to the other things that matter to them. The reality is that HIV touches on a myriad of issues that affect women, from sexuality to parenthood, health care to drug prevention, caretaking to workplace concerns.

Simplistic media portrayals of "risk groups" perpetuate women's sense of false security.

Negotiating for information and safer sex

Safer sex does not happen in a vacuum, but within specific social and cultural contexts. Women's centers can help clients go beyond the advice of brochures to practice safer sex, by dealing with the day-to-day obstacles to prevention. Negotiating for information is a skill that requires practice as well as knowledge. Helping women apply the skills they already have for getting things they want and need in their relationships is a crucial aspect of developing this ability. Community-based organizations can play an important role by doing what they already do so well — helping women to enhance their communication skills through counseling and role plays, learn and practice assertiveness skills, and think through the risks and benefits of raising new sexual and communication issues with their partners.

While many women will need ongoing encouragement for discussing sexual and drug-use histories with their partners, they also need the information, skills, and support to make their own decisions about safer sex and self-protection, regardless of what their partners tell them. Some partners may lie about their past, some may not realize that past sexual and/or drug-related activities have put them at risk, and still others won't remember past experiences that may have placed them at risk. Furthermore, many people have been mislead or had their denial reinforced by media campaigns that downplay the fact that heterosexual sex with a "nice person" can transmit HIV. Simplistic media portrayals of "risk groups" perpetuate women's sense of false security.

In a 1988 study of sexually active people (American Psychological Association, as reported in *The New York Times*, August 14, 1988), 52% of the women interviewed said that asking questions about their partners' drug and sexual histories was one of their main precautions against HIV infection. But 35% of the men in the same study admitted having lied to a woman about their sexual past or drug use in order to have sex with her. Twenty percent of the men said that, in order to have sex with a woman, they would tell her that they had taken the HIV antibody test and had tested negative. This study confirms what common sense would suggest — that asking questions about a partner's sexual and drug history is not a reliable method of protection, not only because people sometimes lie, but because many simply do not realize that they are at risk. Many people infected with HIV do not know they are infected, and few men and women are aware of all their previous partners' sexual and drug-related behavior. So asking questions about a partner's sexual past should be seen as a precaution of minimal value, not as a cornerstone of HIV prevention.

In order to provide meaningful support to clients, it is important to be sensitive to their religious and cultural values and to the difficulty they may face in raising sexual issues with their partners. As advocates for women, our task is to find new ways to work through the many barriers that exist for women who want to protect themselves. Cultural norms can be utilized to enhance education efforts, rather than seen only as obstacles to prevention. For example, in cultures where male protection of the family is a deeply cherished value, safer sex can be framed as a highly desirable way for men to protect their families. Rather than viewing machismo exclusively as a barrier to encouraging heterosexual men to practice safer sex, this cultural framework can be respected without sacrificing the goal of constructive behavioral change.

For women, the practice of safer sex is no simple matter. Aside from the power differential that exists between women and men in all cultures, and which deprives many women of full equality in sexual decision-making, specific cultural and religious obstacles (e.g. prohibitions against condom use or open discussion about sexuality) may also impede a woman's ability to practice safer sex. In *Women and the AIDS Crisis*, author Diane Richardson recounts an episode in which "women were interviewed who were having sexual contact with high-risk men. The majority said that they were afraid of bringing up the issue of safe sex for fear of being rejected, or of the men being unreceptive." Similarly, in their article entitled "Latina Women and AIDS," Dooley Worth and Ruth Rodriguez observed that "Puerto Rican women interviewed in drug treatment programs professed the wish to have their partners use condoms, but felt unable to ask them to do so for fear of being rejected or superceding their defined role."

In addition, many women risk physical, emotional, or economic retaliation from their partners if they insist on condom use. For these women, the long-term risk of HIV disease may seem abstract compared with the real and present chance they take if they anger or alienate their partners. There is also an inherent conflict in the whole notion of safer sex because in many cultures, women's sense of self-worth (or their status within their communities) is closely tied to their

HIV prevention support efforts take time.

role as mothers. The "just say no" approach to HIV prevention, aside from being based on wishful thinking and fostering a phobic attitude toward sexuality, is simply not a viable option for many women. This is why going beyond the superficial level at which most brochures advise about safer sex is so important. Creating programs that improve women's sense of self-worth and empower them to assert their right to health and safety within their relationships is crucial to increasing the acceptance and feasibility of low-risk sex among women and their partners.

A sexual relationship is an interaction between two people, and women cannot bear full responsibility for fostering safer sex in heterosexual relationships. Inroads must be made in reaching men with the safer sex message and with the motivation to share responsibility for condom use — it is, after all, men who wear condoms. In the absence of such a norm among heterosexual men, women's efforts may ultimately prove futile. While our efforts may focus on women's empowerment, we do a disservice if we fail to address the barriers that men's lack of cooperation pose to safer sex efforts. Women's centers can play an important role by helping organizations that reach men (e.g., sports leagues, social clubs, civic groups, churches, etc.) to develop programs in which men can discuss sex roles, learn about HIV, and be encouraged to assume their share of responsibility for protecting their sexual partners and themselves. Programs such as these should not be seen as substitutes for woman-focused prevention efforts, but should occur in tandem with them.

For women, practicing safer sex and getting information about their partners' past behavior may be part of the larger goal of increasing their ability to control their own lives. Given the unequal power dynamic between most men and women, HIV prevention support efforts will inevitably take time. Deeply embedded attitudes and behavior will not change overnight. Service providers should try not to become frustrated if it takes a while to make tangible progress on safer sex issues with women and men, because this process is a vital, albeit labor-intensive one. Our role is to work toward change by providing a framework for support and community-wide education. It helps to remember that many women — of all cultural groups — have successfully struggled to define more equal relationships in which women and men together negotiate for mutually acceptable sexual behavior. These women and men can be important teachers and role models for others.

Safer sex know-how

As important as addressing negotiation issues within the social and cultural contexts that affect sexual communication and decision-making is the need to impart accurate, non-judgmental safer sex information and skills to clients. This does not mean simply promoting condom use in a non-specific way, but rather giving concrete, explicit information about safer sex. Without practical information to back it up, the advice to practice safer sex will ultimately be meaningless to the women you are trying to reach. Sex is an uncomfortable area for many people — including many health educators — so it tends to be "glossed over" in favor of vague recommendations like "use condoms when you have sex." But just as women need information about their bodies in order to take care of their physical health, they also need direct and specific information about sexuality in order to exercise genuine decision making in their sexual lives. Once again, the approaches to conveying this information will vary depending on the needs and values of the women you are working with.

What exactly does it mean to provide explicit safer sex information to your clients? It means, for example, making sure they know that latex (rubber) condoms offer better protection against HIV than "natural" (lambskin) condoms, instead of referring to condoms generically. It means helping them become familiar with condoms, lubricants, and dental dams so that they can feel comfortable about obtaining them, talking about them with partners, and using them correctly. The types of activities you devise to do so can and should be tailored to suit the women you are trying to reach. One popular approach is to arrange at-home small group discussions about safer sex among women. This format is based on "Tupperware Parties" or kitchen table meetings that provide women with forums to meet informally, socialize, and discuss issues of concern to them. Another option is to take a group of the women you serve on an outing to a pharmacy for a "condom shopping expedition" to help them become more knowledgeable about the range of condoms that are available (different styles, sizes, colors, textures, and flavors), to provide support and skills building in overcoming fear or embarrassment when asking for and purchasing them, and to help them begin to associate condoms with pleasure and fun.

In addition to increasing women's overall comfort level around condoms, it is important to provide demonstrations on how to use them properly. Too often, women are "told" to use condoms without being taught (or having their partners taught) how to use them properly. The major cause of condom breakage and failure is incorrect use, so teaching condom use is an integral part of providing meaningful HIV prevention information. There are some good videos available on safer sex which include condom demonstrations (look for the ones with a sense of humor), but best of all are in-person demonstrations by people who are knowledgeable about safer sex and can convey a sense of comfort and ease in discussing these issues. Lots of safer sex trainers use a banana or anatomical model, and some involve participants in "put the condom on the banana" contests or races to help them get used to handling condoms, as well as to create a more relaxed and positive attitude toward safer sex. This is all part of the work of helping people overcome their negative associations with condoms and the resistance to safer sex practices that result from these feelings.

Women also need to know about dental dams, which are often the "forgotten" element of the safer sex education. Dental dams are thin squares of latex about 6" x 6" that can be used as HIV-prevention barriers during oral sex on women. Dental dams, as the name suggests, are used during dental procedures. However, because of their size, thinness, and the fact that no other type of barrier was (or is) available on the market for oral sex on women, ingenious HIV educators came up with the idea of using dental dams. Because dams, like condoms, are made of latex, they are thought to work in the same way to prevent vaginal secretions and/or menstrual blood from passing from a woman's vagina to her partner's mouth. By allowing for women's sexual pleasure and enjoyment in the context of HIV prevention, they provide an important counterpart to condoms.

Unfortunately, however, dental dams do have some caveats: they are often hard to obtain (dental or medical supply houses sometimes carry them, and some HIV/AIDS organizations distribute them); many people find them cumbersome and difficult to use; they were not originally intended for safer sex purposes and are therefore not specially designed as such; and no empirical testing has been done on their efficacy as barriers to HIV transmission during oral sex. Even taking these negatives into account, dental dams are one of the few options available for women wishing to continue enjoying oral sex "safely." An alternative to the use of dental dams is to cut an unlubricated latex condom lengthwise and open it up to form a "homemade" dam. The use of plastic food wrap in lieu of cut condoms or dental dams is controversial, both because such products may contain toxic chemicals and because they have not been scientifically tested as barriers against the virus.

Lubricant is another important safer sex topic that sometimes gets lost in superficial discussions of safer sex. While many people know that condoms prevent transmission of HIV, most are unaware that their choice of lubricants can either enhance or defeat their efforts to have sex without transmitting HIV. Your clients need to know that commonly used oil-based lubricants like Crisco, Vaseline, hand lotion, baby oil, and grease break down the latex in condoms, causing them to weaken, and compromising their capacity to prevent HIV transmission. Water-based lubricants like KY jelly are recommended because they do not damage condoms. The use of lubricants containing the spermicide Nonoxynol-9 has also been recommended since this chemical has been found to kill HIV in the test tube. However, some people are allergic to Nonoxynol-9, so this is not an option for everyone.

Women's centers and other CBOs can routinely make in-depth safer sex information available to their clients in a climate which encourages questions and the open discussion of experience and exchange of information. The silence that surrounds sexuality works against the promotion of risk reduction because it reinforces sexual ignorance, shame, and fear. An effective prevention approach will stress sexual empowerment and increased awareness about the body, sexuality, and risk reduction techniques. Such efforts must occur within the context of cultural taboos against the discussion of sex. Although this is not an easy line to walk, it is important to balance the desire to communicate HIV prevention information to women with the need to convey this knowledge in a manner that is acceptable to them.

5

Key Issues for Women

For every woman at risk of becoming *infected* with HIV, there are countless others who are or will be *affected* by the AIDS crisis. This chapter provides an overview of some of the different ways the epidemic may impact upon the women you serve. Topics addressed include: stages of HIV infection and illness, HIV antibody testing and counseling, reproductive issues, women and drugs, violence against women, and parental issues.

Stages of HIV infection and illness

When we talk about AIDS, we are really talking about a spectrum of illness in which the immune system of a person infected with HIV is progressively weakened. As shown in Figure 3 on the next page, this continuum includes infected persons who have no symptoms (also known as "asymptomatic"), persons who have a range of minor or serious symptoms related to immune compromise that fall short of the clinical definition for AIDS, and persons with "full-blown" AIDS, which represents the most advanced stage of the progressive depletion of the body's defense system. HIV-positive people who have one or more specific cancers, opportunistic infections (life-threatening illnesses which only occur when the immune system is damaged), dementia, or wasting syndrome are categorized by the federal Centers for Disease Control (CDC) as having Acquired Immune Deficiency Syndrome, or AIDS. At the beginning of the epidemic, these categories were seen as separate and rigid stages of illness, but now experts treat the syndrome as a continuum of HIV-related illnesses, ranging from HIV infection to the final stages of CDC-defined AIDS.

Emotional responses to HIV infection and illness

Individuals who first discover they have HIV-related illness or who have tested positive for HIV antibodies, often experience a combination of shock, denial, fear, anger, anxiety, depression, and a sense of isolation. In addition to facing a potentially fatal illness, they must cope with having a disease that has been highly stigmatized as a result of prejudices associated with IV drug use and homosexuality. Since HIV disease is seen by many people as a punishment for behavior of which they do not approve, it is not surprising that people with HIV often face rejection and abandonment by their loved ones. Because of the misinformation and stigma that surrounds this illness, those affected need not only medical and practical assistance, but emotional support and a sense of community. Community-based organizations can help create a context of caring for people who are facing HIV

Figure #3:   <u>**The Spectrum of HIV Disease**</u>

The bar below represents the continuum of HIV infection and disease. When a person becomes infected with HIV, the virus slowly weakens his or her immune system. The time from infection to full-blown AIDS is approximately ten years, although it varies greatly from person to person. The chronology below is not the same for every person either —some persons move from asymptomatic directly to AIDS, while others progress incrementally along the full spectrum.

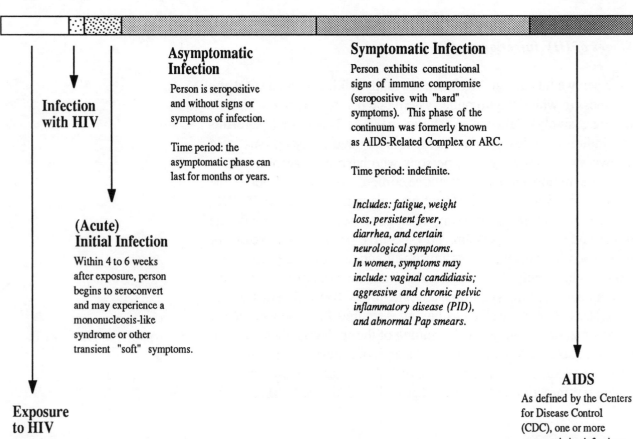

Asymptomatic Infection

Person is seropositive and without signs or symptoms of infection.

Time period: the asymptomatic phase can last for months or years.

Infection with HIV

(Acute) Initial Infection

Within 4 to 6 weeks after exposure, person begins to seroconvert and may experience a mononucleosis-like syndrome or other transient "soft" symptoms.

Symptomatic Infection

Person exhibits constitutional signs of immune compromise (seropositive with "hard" symptoms). This phase of the continuum was formerly known as AIDS-Related Complex or ARC.

Time period: indefinite.

Includes: fatigue, weight loss, persistent fever, diarrhea, and certain neurological symptoms. In women, symptoms may include: vaginal candidiasis; aggressive and chronic pelvic inflammatory disease (PID), and abnormal Pap smears.

Exposure to HIV

Indefinite number of exposures can lead to infection. (A person can be exposed one time and get infected, or be exposed 100 times and remain uninfected -- each exposure is unique.)

AIDS

As defined by the Centers for Disease Control (CDC), one or more opportunistic infections, cancers, neurological diseases, or wasting syndrome. Includes persons who are minimally symptomatic as well as those who are very ill.

Time period: indefinite.

Includes: dementia, lymphomas, and such opportunistic infections as Pneumocystis carinii pneumonia (PCP), toxoplasmosis, cytomegalovirus, and oral and esophageal candidiasis (thrush), among others.

illness in their own lives or the lives of those they love. This can include sponsoring support groups, social events, "drop-in" centers, meal programs, special outings, and other activities. If possible, it should also involve the creation of support systems for partners, friends, and families.

Discrimination

Along with the personal loss of support from friends and family that may follow a positive HIV antibody test result or an AIDS diagnosis, many people also face the wider, systemic problem of discrimination. Discrimination in insurance, health care facilities, housing, employment, public accomodations, prisons, and schools is still very much a reality for people with HIV disease, even though in many communities such discrimination is illegal. The recently passed Americans With Disabilities Act forbids discrimination on the basis of HIV infection on a nationwide level, and will take effect in 1992. Nevertheless, discrimination will continue, and must be monitored and fought. Your center can identify discrimination cases that might otherwise go undiscovered and unresolved. You can help clients to understand and pursue their rights through the legal channels available in your region and through advocacy for implementation of nondiscriminatory policies. Developing good working relationships with local AIDS advocates and civil rights organizations is an intrinsic aspect of providing meaningful support to people with HIV disease, many of whom will face discrimination of one sort or another during the course of their illness.

Aside from its devastating impact on individuals and families, discrimination hinders efforts to curb the epidemic by creating a punitive environment that drives those who most need help "underground," making it difficult for them to seek information, acknowledge their own risk, and take appropriate action to protect themselves and others. Women's centers and other CBOs can address discrimination by providing community-wide education to improve community attitudes, testifying on behalf of compassionate regulations at legislative or civil rights hearings, and helping people with HIV disease to understand and secure their rights.

Impact on women

As discussed throughout this guide, there are many ways in which the impact of HIV on women differs from that on men. One important difference is that women are frequently more isolated during their illness. Women's traditional social role as caregivers means that women with HIV disease may put their own health needs after those of their partners and children, often to the point of failing to get medical attention until their own health has seriously deteriorated. Even more significant is the fact that the vast majority of women affected have little or no access to quality health care. Lack of access to housing and health and supportive services increases the day-to-day stress in these women's lives and decreases their chances of long-term survival. These health and psychosocial needs are not likely to be met by traditional avenues of health care, nor are such women likely to seek help from institutions that have historically failed to meet their needs. It is in precisely this area, then, that grass roots community-based organizations who *have* earned the community's trust can play a key role by addressing some of the special problems faced by women with HIV disease. Creating support systems for women, acting as advocates for quality health care and related services, advocating for increased participation of women in promising experimental treatment protocols, developing gender-specific HIV-related services, and providing prevention information on a range of HIV-related topics of concern to women are a few examples of important ways women's centers can help.

> **The majority of women with HIV illness have little access to quality health care.**

The "Worried Well"

Another group of women you may be working with are known as the "worried well." These are women who are currently in good health, but who are concerned that they may have been exposed to HIV. They may have chosen not to take the HIV antibody test for various reasons, or they may still be deciding whether or not to get tested. "Worried well" support groups are for women who are uncertain of their health status, but who want to take some kind of action *now* on behalf of their mental and physical health.

Support groups for such women generally focus on health maintenance, risk assessment, concrete information about HIV, exploration of feelings and fears, practical support, decision-making regarding the HIV antibody test, and on helping women confront illness issues while they are still healthy.

HIV antibody testing and counseling

HIV antibody testing is a complex and controversial issue, and one which people are likely to raise at your center once you begin addressing HIV/AIDS issues. It is important to understand how the test works and what it does. The following section on HIV counseling and testing provides only a basic overview of some of the main issues to be aware of. More detailed information on HIV antibody testing is available through some of the AIDS organizations listed in Appendix B.

Taking the test

The HIV antibody test has been one of the most heated issues of debate both within and outside of the communities impacted by the epidemic. The HIV antibody test is often referred to in "shorthand" as "the AIDS test." This is a misnomer, however, because the test does not tell whether someone has AIDS. This phrase (though widely used by the mass media and general public) is discouraged by HIV educators because it creates the misleading impression that having the human immunodeficiency virus inside one's body is the same as having AIDS.

The HIV antibody test indicates whether a person's body has marshalled an attack against an "invasion" by HIV by creating antibodies. The test only detects HIV antibodies, not the virus itself. A positive HIV antibody test means that a person has gotten HIV into her/his body. The test does *not* tell if or when a person will get AIDS.

Some people who are infected will test negative because it normally takes anywhere between three weeks and 18 months (and in some cases up to three years) after infection for the body to develop antibodies. This means that a woman infected two months prior to testing might test negative because her body has not yet developed the antibodies that the test identifies. People whose immune systems are compromised due to drug or alcohol abuse or other immunosuppressive diseases (e.g. cancer or lupus), may take even longer to produce antibodies since their immune systems are already impaired and may therefore marshall slower responses to invasion.

Some women who are worried about the possibility of being infected, or who are certain that past behavior has put them at risk, may choose to get tested. There are many good reasons to get tested — especially with the advent of better treatment options over the past couple of years — but the test has limitations and potential liabilities, as well. Some women will want to reduce their anxiety by knowing one way or the other whether they are infected, and the test is a good — though not foolproof — way to find that out. Early medical intervention in persons infected with HIV is a very important weapon

Early medical intervention is a very important weapon against HIV disease.

against HIV disease. And the value of early intervention increases as more and more effective experimental treatments become available. The key is making sure the women you serve will have *access* to these medical options if they test positive.

While the value of getting tested has increased significantly since the days when the test first became available, the decision to take it is a personal one; emotional devastation, discrimination, and lack of access to treatment, support, and resources still weigh heavily for many people on the "other side" of the testing debate. There is no "right" or "wrong" answer for everybody. Individuals needs to decide whether and when they want to know, and should receive as much information as possible about the measures they can take to protect their health regardless of their decision. As a service provider, it is important to be well informed about testing and services, so that you can support your clients in making informed decisions based upon the most current information available and individual situations. This means being able to explain complex issues in a way that will be clear to those you serve. And it means supporting them in making the decisions that they feel are best for them.

Testing negative

A negative HIV antibody test result means that no HIV antibodies were detected in the person's blood sample. Because of the virus' long incubation period, a negative test result is of limited meaning, however, if the client has recently engaged in high-risk behavior. It means even less if one continues to engage in unsafe sex or unsafe IV drug use, since a negative test result does not guarantee that one will remain uninfected in the future. This is why it is so important that all testing be accompanied by extensive counseling to help people understand the test's parameters and to help them keep from getting infected (or reinfected) in the future. Regardless of whether a person tests negative or positive, the basic message is the same: practice safer sex, and if you use IV drugs, clean your injection paraphernalia.

Testing positive

A positive test result means that HIV antibodies were detected in the person's blood sample and that the person is infected with HIV. While a positive test result is never welcome news, persons who are emotionally prepared may feel empowered by the knowledge of their status and be motivated to try to access existing treatments and promising experimental therapies. It may also help provide the impetus to begin other activities that will improve their health, such as eating right, getting adequate rest and exercise, and practicing risk reduction in their sexual and drug activities. On the emotional front, knowledge of one's health status may encourage the reaching out for support in one's personal life, and through existing services and networks for people with HIV.

It is important to understand, however, that most people take the test hoping that they will test negative. For those who get a positive result, the test — especially initially — may be more immobilizing than empowering, and for some, the fear and anger produced by a positive test result will precipitate a period of crisis that requires intervention. This is why it is vital to offer extensive pre-test counseling to help women think through their reactions to receiving either a positive or negative result, decide whether and how to elicit support from family and friends, assess potential legal and discrimination issues that may result from learning the test result, and consider whether knowing their test results will lead them to reduce or increase risk-taking or unhealthy behavior. Working through these issues *before* getting tested makes the test a more useful health promotion tool and increases its capacity to expand the individual's health options, rather than narrow them.

HIV counseling

One issue to consider in pre-test counseling is whether the woman already has strong personal support, be it partner, family, or friends. Getting tested might have a dramatic impact on this support system. Would her supports remain if she tested positive, or would they collapse? What kinds of backup assistance can be put into place for her *before* she gets tested? Though many friends and families are extremely supportive of people who become sick with HIV disease, some will react out of ignorance because they themselves have not been reached with accurate, credible information and support.

Consider to what extent the woman can obtain the services and support she will need once she has received her test result. If she tests positive, will she be able to gain access to AZT and the other prophylactic treatments that are now available? If she wishes to do so, does she have the means to improve her diet, the time to exercise, the transportation to get to a support group? Will the people in her life encourage her to make and sustain such changes? Are substance abuse treatment services available to her if she needs them? If appropriate services are not accessible to her, will knowing her test result help her? Some experts argue that taking the test helps to motivate HIV-positive people to practice safer sex, while others point out that knowledge does not automatically lead to behavioral change. For some people, a positive test result will provide impetus for making personal changes, while others (especially those with few external support systems or those in early recovery from drug or alcohol abuse) may feel unable to change, or that their life is more unmanageable than before. As many people who do AIDS work have observed, safer sex and safer drug practices should be adopted by *all* people who feel they may be at risk, regardless of the result of their antibody test. Part of the counseling that should follow all testing involves helping people address issues of behavioral change. If the person has tested positive, post-test counseling may also offer emotional support, practical information, and help with arranging for appropriate medical intervention, social services, psychosocial support, and other areas in which the individual may need help.

There can also be legal and discrimination-related ramifications for people who take the HIV antibody test, and being aware of these can help the women you serve make fully informed decisions about whether and how to get tested. Laws and regulations regarding confidentiality, partner notification, and protection from HIV-related discrimination differ throughout the United States. These regulations are constantly changing. Staying in contact with state and local AIDS services, advocacy, and legal rights organizations will help you keep apprised of laws that may affect your clients. Informing women who want to take the test of the possible effects of local regulations and of their rights is an important part of helping them make beneficial decisions.

There is also a political aspect to the debates that surround the test. Many women's health and AIDS advocates have observed that women of color are increasingly the targets of campaigns encouraging people to be tested, yet their communities rarely receive priority in terms of support services and education. HIV counseling and testing is increasingly being offered at family planning and health clinics. Since it is primarily poor, young women of color who use these clinics, this kind of targeting — particularly in the absence of education, quality health care, services, and follow-up — is seen by many advocates as problematic. Some question the professed commitment to testing people without providing the range of services that those who have tested positive will require. They question the purpose of testing people without having a plan for their care once the results are known. Your center can advocate for increased services to communities at risk, support the availability of anonymous testing and high-quality pre- and post-test counseling, and work toward educating your community about the personal and political issues that surround the decision to get tested, the ways testing policies are carried out, and the availability of HIV-related medical services and resources.

Women of color are often targeted for HIV testing, but rarely receive priority in terms of services and support.

Anonymous vs. confidential testing

An important distinction to be aware of is the difference between "anonymous" and "confidential" testing. Anonymous testing allows people to get tested without giving any identifying information whatsoever. Instead of giving their real name, they are given a code number as an identifier. Anonymous testing eliminates the risk that others will know a person's test result unless she/he chooses to tell them.

With confidential testing, a woman gives her name, but the test results are considered private. However, confidential testing is not fool proof, and there have been cases where the confidentiality of the test result was breached by a health care practitioner or someone else who had access to the information. Under certain circumstances, confidential information may also be legally obtained by health professionals, insurance companies, and other agencies. Because of the possibility of breaches in confidential testing, many HIV/AIDS advocates have pressed for the availability of anonymous testing in order to give people the option of getting tested while retaining control over how that information is shared.

Reproductive issues

Because HIV can be passed from mother to child during pregnancy and childbirth, and possibly through breastfeeding, it has a profound impact on a range of reproductive issues, including childbearing and child-raising, abortion, sterilization, and how family planning counseling is conducted. The epidemic poses new challenges for those struggling on behalf of women's right to make informed, independent decisions about their reproductive options. Women's centers and women's health advocates can help insure that during this epidemic, these rights are not further abridged. Programs providing family planning services can integrate information about risk reduction into their current counseling activities, and can make sure the women they serve are aware of the fact that among birth control techniques, only condoms can significantly reduce HIV transmission.

Pregnancy, women, and HIV

We hear a lot about babies who are born infected with HIV and who later develop AIDS. A baby born infected with HIV is born of a mother who is also infected. All babies born to infected women will test HIV positive for the first 12 to 15 months of their lives because they are born with their mothers' antibodies, which they retain until they develop their own after about a year. Some babies born to infected mothers will turn out to be HIV negative once they have developed their own antibodies; an estimated 30% will turn out to be infected. Therefore, testing a newborn only reveals the mother's HIV antibody status for certain — unless the infant is also exhibiting symptoms of illness. Many women learn of their own HIV infection as a result of giving birth to an HIV positive asymptomatic or ill child.

The growing number of pediatric cases of HIV disease raises controversial questions, including those involving "boarder babies," foster care, and the presence of children with HIV in the schools. There has also been debate about "the right" of HIV positive women to have children. It has been suggested — both implicitly and explicitly — that women not currently pregnant, but known to have HIV disease should be discouraged from becoming pregnant in the future. Various governmental agencies have recommended that HIV and family planning counselors tell high-risk women to postpone pregnancy "until more is known or there is a cure."

It used to be thought that pregnancy could accelerate the progression of HIV disease in asymptomatic infected women, and this was seen as an important reason for discouraging pregnancy in the interests of the woman's health. However, current research suggests that pregnancy does not increase the risk of accelerated progression of illness. Most discussion of the risks associated with HIV and pregnancy have therefore focused exclusively on the health of the baby.

From the viewpoint of empowering women and their communities, there are several important problems with recommendations to "avoid" pregnancy, however well-intentioned they may appear. First, such recommendations often highlight the tragedy of HIV-infected babies. They show little or no concern for their mothers, presenting women's needs only insofar as they relate to their reproductive capacities. Second, they occur in a context where HIV education for women at risk is still minimal at best. Third, this approach limits women's rights to make their own reproductive decisions. As stated earlier, a woman who is HIV positive has about a 30% chance of giving birth to an infected baby. For a woman living in a community with high rates of infant morbidity and mortality, this may seem like relatively good odds for having a healthy baby. For some women, the fear of becoming sick and dying is eased by the chance of having a child that will live a long and healthy life. For many HIV-positive women who see their options diminishing in so many other ways, the choice of whether or not to bear a child is vital to maintaining a sense of control over the ability to determine the course of their lives. Finally, the recommendation that HIV-positive women "just say no" to having a child runs contrary to most religious and cultural belief systems, in which childbearing is presented as an intrinsic part of women's role and a major way in which her identity is defined. The limits HIV can place on a woman's reproductive life can have devastating social and emotional consequences for her.

Some service providers may feel uneasy about a woman's decision to keep or abort an at-risk fetus; nevertheless, that decision is the woman's alone. Non-directive counseling for an HIV-positive pregnant woman, or one considering pregnancy, can help her make an informed decision by presenting all possible options and exploring the potential consequences of each, including, for example, what arrangements she would make for the baby if she became too ill to care for it, and who would raise the child if she died. Some service providers take their HIV-positive clients to a hospital to see babies with AIDS, not to dissuade them from having children, but to give them a realistic understanding of what raising a sick child might be like. It is also important to support the woman's empowerment in advocating for herself within the medical and social service systems that she will encounter during her pregnancy and throughout her illness. Presenting viable options includes providing her with information about appropriate medical issues, community resources, and linkages with support services.

Once a woman has made up her mind about whether or not to keep her baby, she should be able to count on receiving support from the service providers she works with, regardless of whether or not her decision coincides with their own beliefs.

Non-directive counseling means laying out all the options and exploring the consequences of each.

Abortion, discrimination, and HIV

Since many women's centers and health agencies provide (or offer referrals to) family planning and abortion services, it is important to be aware of an emerging discrimination issue which uniquely impacts women: the denial of abortion services to women who are HIV-positive. Although HIV-infected individuals may be victims of broad-based discrimination when pursuing routine medical and dental care, the issue of HIV discrimination in abortion services is particularly ironic since women with HIV disease often seek abortions in order to avoid bearing infected children.

A 1990 study conducted by the New York City Commission on Human Rights revealed that 20% of abortion clinics in New York City turned away women who indicated that they were HIV positive. Although a variety of reasons were offered for such policies, there is no medical basis for denying services to HIV-positive women.

Women's centers and other community organizations who provide referrals for family planning and/or abortion services can and should make sure that such services will be available to women without regard to their HIV status. Discrimination prevention usually entails a balance of education and legal recourse. Programs such as yours can work with local civil rights and anti-discrimination programs to help monitor the availability of all health and reproductive services for HIV infected women, and can also educate service providers. If your agency provides family planning or abortion services, make sure all appropriate staff are fully aware of the universal blood precautions issued by the federal government which should be followed with *all* clients, whether or not they are thought or known to be HIV positive. Staff should also be offered support in dealing with their feelings and fears about providing services to HIV-positive clients.

Artificial insemination

Another important reproductive issue is artificial (or alternative) insemination (AI), to which a few cases of HIV disease among women have been linked. Most women seeking to be artificially inseminated use a sperm bank or a private physician. Although most licensed sperm banks now screen for HIV, the donor screening guidelines established by the American Fertility Society and the American Association of Tissue Banks are completely voluntary. And according to a 1988 report by the Congressional Office of Technology Assessment (OTA), less than half of physicians regularly doing AI test donors for HIV antibodies. Since neither sperm banks nor physicians are mandated to screen donors, it is important for women to be "educated consumers" when seeking these services. Women using a "home donor" should be strongly encouraged to ask about his risk factors, and to speak with him about the possibility of getting tested before donating. The CDC has established guidelines for screening donors prior to artificial insemination. Detailed discussions of how to do safer AI can be found in some of the materials listed in Appendix A.

Women and drugs

Both directly and indirectly, drug use is the major cause of HIV infection among women. There are several connections between women, drugs, and HIV infection that are important to understand if your organization is planning to become involved in HIV issues. This section briefly discusses the major linkages, including women's primary and secondary risks from intravenous (IV) needle-sharing drug use, the impact of the crack epidemic, the effect of alcohol and other drugs, drug treatment issues, and barriers to drug and HIV prevention.

Intravenous drug use

The most important link between women and HIV is the risk to women who share contaminated intravenous (IV) needles and other equipment to shoot heroin, cocaine, or speed. IV equipment that has been shared usually retains a small amount of blood. The next person who uses that equipment will inject some of that blood directly into their bloodstream along with the drug they are taking. If the first person using the equipment is infected, those sharing the needle are at high risk of becoming infected. Because sharing IV needles and other equipment involves a direct route of blood-to-blood contact, it is one of the most efficient modes of HIV transmission. With well over half of all IV drug users in New York City estimated to be infected with HIV, the risk from sharing IV drug equipment is, in many areas, extremely high. Over half of all U.S. AIDS cases among women are the result of sharing unclean injection equipment with infected persons.

Unprotected sex with intravenous drug users

The second highest cause of HIV infection among women is unprotected sexual contact with partners who have engaged in intravenous needle-sharing behavior. The vast majority of women who were infected with HIV through unprotected heterosexual intercourse were infected by men who shared IV needles or equipment. Some women who became infected this way had no idea that they were at risk, either because they were unaware of their sexual partner's current IV drug use or because their partner had used IV drugs in the past. Other women were aware of their partner's past or current high-risk activities, but felt unable to advocate for safer sex practices in their relationships.

Women, AIDS, and the crack epidemic

An increasingly important dynamic in the spread of HIV is the crack epidemic. Crack is a highly purified, highly addictive, smokable form of cocaine. In the United States, hundreds of thousands of persons are believed to be addicted to crack. In the early stages of their addiction, people who smoke crack experience periods of heightened sexual activity and disinhibition, often leading to repeated sexual encounters without the use of condoms. The crack epidemic has impacted young women more heavily than other drug epidemics. In crack houses — where crack is sold and smoked — women often barter for the drug with sex, or have sex to get money to buy more crack. Because the crack high is brief, women crack addicts may engage in unprotected sex for drugs many times each day with multiple partners. These partners may be infected with HIV through sharing IV equipment or participating in other high-risk behaviors. This dynamic means that crack is becoming an increasingly significant route of HIV transmission for women.

Crack is becoming a significant route of HIV transmission for women.

Alcohol and other drugs

When we talk about drug use and HIV, the connection seems obvious. However, alcohol often does not come to mind in these discussions. There are two important links between alcohol use and HIV. First, alcohol impairs judgment and removes inhibitions, which increases people's likelihood of engaging in high-risk behavior. A person who has had a few drinks may not be as resolute about using a condom as someone who is sober. Second, alcohol is an immune suppressant, which can have serious consequences for persons who are infected with HIV and whose immune systems are already in jeopardy. It is important to realize that, although legally sanctioned and socially acceptable, alcohol is a powerful and addictive drug, in terms of its immediate impact, the ways in which it is used and abused, and its long-term health consequences. Other drugs may also tax the immune system and make people more prone to engaging in high-risk behaviors that they would otherwise avoid.

Treatment programs

If you are working with women who want to go into treatment for their drug problems, you may find the there is a lack of programs to refer them to. This problem may be exacerbated if your client is pregnant or has children. Although the idea of funding drug treatment is now regaining legitimacy as part of the "war on drugs," there is a severe shortage of such facilities in the United States and a continued lack of strong economic and political support for the development of new programs. It is estimated that at any one time, existing programs are able to treat fewer than 150,000 of the estimated 1.2 million IV drug users in America. This does not include persons who abuse drugs other than those taken intravenously. Budget cuts, lack of political support, and community opposition to proposed drug treatment programs have been cited as the major reasons for the shortage. In many areas, treatment programs have waiting lists of up to six months. "Free treatment on demand" is a long way off for persons seeking help with their drug problems in communities throughout the U.S.

Treatment programs using models which are appropriate for women and which provide childcare are even more scarce. If you are planning to refer women with children to drug treatment, be advised that few programs will allow women to take children. These clients will be faced with a choice between receiving treatment and remaining with their children. Advocacy is needed to insure that drug treatment is available on demand and that existing drug treatment programs are accessible to women. Supportive groups like Cocaine Anonymous (CA), Narcotics Anonymous (NA), and Alcoholics Anonymous (AA) can be important alternatives for women who cannot access or are not ready to go into treatment.

Providing education

All women who use drugs — whether or not they are planning to stop — are entitled to receive the information and support they need to protect themselves from HIV infection. Teaching IV drug-using women how to disinfect their injection equipment with bleach or rubbing alcohol, although politically controversial, is an important way to help them stay alive long enough to be able to get off drugs in the future.

Providing women who are using other kinds of drugs or who are the sexual partners of IV drug users with support and information about safer sex is another important aspect of working with women who are impacted by the twin epidemics of drug use and HIV infection. Remember to highlight the risk involved in taking *any* drug, along with the direct risk related to sharing IV equipment.

Barriers to HIV prevention

The barriers to HIV prevention among women are many, but they may seem especially daunting with respect to drug-addicted women. Fear of addicts (addictophobia) and the belief that addicts can be easily identified (stereotyping) both hinder efforts to get important prevention information to women who use drugs. To overcome these problems, staff training by experts on drug-related issues and a policy of providing the full range of HIV prevention information to all clients is advised.

Staff training will help reduce service providers' fear of

clients who use drugs, and will enable them to convey important risk reduction information to these women in a non-judgmental and supportive manner. Training will also help to challenge stereotypic attitudes regarding addicts and drug users. It will help providers understand that women whose lives are impacted by drugs are not always easily identified. They are not necessarily spending their lives in crack houses or "shooting galleries" (places where IV drugs and equipment are sold and used). Many women at risk are maintaining lifestyles that would not seem to suggest that drugs are part of their lives. They come from every socio-economic group. Some use drugs recreationally, or only on occasion, and are not addicted. Their need for information and support around safer drug use may not always be apparent to service providers, but it is nonetheless very real.

HIV and violence against women

Domestic violence

Women's centers and other programs working on issues of domestic violence are facing a range of HIV-related questions and concerns as more of their clients find themselves (and their families) impacted by the epidemic.

In contemplating how HIV might affect the domestic violence services offered by your agency, draw upon any past HIV-related experience your program has gained, and try to anticipate scenarios that might occur in the future. The following are just a few examples of the types of situations which might arise:

> ☐ A domestic violence survivor finds out that her partner is HIV positive or reveals to a counselor that her partner is an active IV drug user;
>
> ☐ The volunteers at a local safe house for battered women inform your program that they will not accept referrals of women with AIDS;
>
> ☐ While in a shelter, a woman's child is diagnosed as having HIV infection;
>
> ☐ A member of your battered women's support group "comes out" as HIV positive to the group, and several members refuse to attend the next meeting because they don't want to "catch" AIDS.

In trying to prepare for such situations, think about their impact on the services you offer, your internal policies and protocols, and the needs of staff. Consider what can be done immediately and over the long term to insure that you will be prepared to assist clients facing both domestic violence and HIV-related concerns.

As with so many other HIV-related issues, the first step is often allaying the fears of staff and clients. Start with HIV training and support for your staff and volunteers. The training will allow them to air their concerns and help them to feel more competent and comfortable in dealing with clients with HIV disease or related problems. Once they feel able to address the issues, they can go on to work with clients who are directly impacted, and to provide appropriate AIDS education to others.

The next step is to develop policies and protocols within your organization addressing such issues as confidentiality, prevention of HIV discrimination, and adherence to state and local regulations regarding testing, privacy, and civil rights.

You will also need to look at your programs and consider the types of support structures (psychosocial, medical, legal, etc.) that might be developed or enhanced to better serve HIV-positive battered women and/or children. What will your long-term and emergency shelter and housing programs need either on-site or by referral to meet the special needs of such women and their children? What kinds of educational activities will other clients need — both in terms of co-existing with HIV-positive women and families, and with respect to future prevention?

Building linkages is critical. How can your in-house referral system be enhanced to improve clients' access to outside support systems? What new interagency linkages can be made or what current referral sources can be enhanced? Will relations with new agencies need to be developed to enhance your advocacy activities? How can your organization help outside groups to better meet the needs of your clients?

Some organizations providing domestic violence services have already begun to address these issues. Their experiences may be useful in helping your agency to develop new programs or resources, train staff, integrate "HIV consciousness" into existing programs, create appropriate policies internally, and advocate for clients in other arenas. Your state task force on domestic violence may also be important sources of support and assistance (see Appendix A for a list of resources on this emerging issue).

For nearly two decades, battered women's counselors and advocates have worked with an empowerment model which supports women in protecting their health and well-being by surviving and moving beyond abusive situations. These individuals and agencies have much to offer those who are engaged in the long-term and labor-intensive work of helping women to practice safer sex and adopt new behaviors to protect themselves from HIV.

Sexual assault

As with domestic violence programs, agencies providing services to rape survivors will benefit from increasing their knowledge about HIV generally and then examining the specific ways that the epidemic might impact on the work they do. Here are a few scenarios that such agencies might face:

> ❑ A rape survivor wants to take the HIV antibody test immediately after the assault to find out if she "got AIDS" from the rapist;
>
> ❑ A woman who was raped by her boyfriend tells the counselor that she thinks he has AIDS;
>
> ❑ The local hospital asks for your agency's help in developing a new HIV testing policy for rape survivors that come to their emergency room;
>
> ❑ A local prosecutor urges your client to demand that the defendant in a sexual assault case be ordered by the court to have an HIV antibody test;
>
> ❑ In a staff meeting, counselors raise the concern that their clients are increasingly focusing on possible HIV infection to the exclusion of other aspects of the assault.

Once again, key areas to address are staff training, program enhancement, client education, internal policy/protocol, network and referral building, and legal or political advocacy.

The varied issues raised by the intersection of sexual assault and HIV are among the most complex raised by the epidemic. Agencies that provide services to rape survivors will need to take time and care in developing responses to these emerging issues. In thinking about these problems, it will quickly become clear that there are no easy answers. The following is a basic outline of the major areas of concern related to HIV and sexual assault: counseling, legal, and medical issues. It is intended to help stimulate your thinking about how these issues might affect your work and some of the things you can do to address them.

Counseling issues

Counselors will need extensive education in order to provide sensitive counseling and accurate information to clients (and their partners or families) about: the potential risk of HIV transmission through sexual assault in general; the specific risk based on the particular circumstances of each case (the nature and duration of the assault, whether or not the perpetrator's health status was known to the victim, etc.); HIV antibody testing; and the impact on future or current sexual relationships. Clients will also need help coping with assault-related issues that are exacerbated by concerns about HIV: for instance, feelings of toxicity and stigma associated with both rape and HIV infection, and the need to discuss the assault and its possible HIV-related implications with partners or lovers. Counselors should also be aware that fear of HIV sometimes masks anxieties related to the assault, and will need to both address their clients' AIDS-related concerns, and help them focus on the process of recovering from the assault itself. To supplement your counseling efforts, you may want to develop special print materials on sexual assault and HIV for both clients and service providers, and to include some basic HIV information in your "general" print materials.

Legal and policy issues

The court system is becoming increasingly involved with a range of sexual assault and HIV issues, from mandatory testing of defendants to the admissibility of a victim's HIV antibody status at the time of the assault. These are complicated issues and laws vary from state to state. You can assist your clients by finding out how local laws and policies might affect them, and then communicating this information to them. Sexual assault advocates and women's centers, traditionally aligned with civil liberties causes, are now negotiating new ground in deciding where to come down with regard to mandatory testing of sexual assault defendants and other issues. Some organizations have published guidelines and reports (see Appendix A) on the new and developing legal, medical, and psychosocial problems related to sexual assault and HIV, and some statewide sexual assault networks are helping their member organizations to address these concerns.

Medical issues and HIV antibody testing

Throughout the country, hospital emergency rooms are responding to women's concerns about HIV transmission as a result of an assault. Some physicians offer victims the HIV antibody test when they are first admitted for emergency room treatment, but because of the virus' incubation period, taking the test at that point will only reveal a woman's antibody status at the time of the rape, rather than indicating whether she was infected as a result of it. Your program can provide a valuable service by lending its expertise with sexual assault issues to local hospitals and medical providers as they begin to define their policies on HIV counseling, testing, and medical intervention for rape survivors. Such protocols should take into account any legal ramifications related to HIV testing and how they might affect the court cases of clients wishing to file charges. In addition to advocating for appropriate protocols in other settings, counselors and volunteers will need to know about these issues in order to provide competent counsel and advice to clients in need.

Women are the primary care-takers in our society.

Women as caregivers

An important aspect of the epidemic that receives little attention outside of HIV social service circles is the issue of the women who care for people with HIV disease, whether the setting is institutional or in the home. Women are — on both the personal and professional levels — the primary caretakers of families and the sick in our society. Because women make up the vast majority of social workers, nurses, nurses' aides, and home health care workers, they are often at the "frontline" of dealing with persons with HIV illness. A comprehensive view of the impact of HIV on women necessitates addressing the way in which caregivers are affected. Issues to consider include: the psychological effect upon women whose paid work now brings them into contact with the mortality of a great number of their peers or persons younger than themselves; women performing unpaid caregiving functions in communities that are being devastated by the epidemic; and women who themselves have HIV infection or disease and must continue caring for (possibly sick) partners, children, and/or other family members.

The HIV epidemic intersects with socio-economic factors and women's societal roles to create additional hardships for low-income women and their families. Because women are often the heads of households and/or the primary economic support in low-income families, and because women in general are paid significantly less than men, poor women and their families are particularly vulnerable to the effects of this epidemic. In addition, most women who provide care to people with HIV disease on a paid basis tend to be recruited from communities that are heavily impacted by the epidemic, as well as by other social hardships.

Women's centers and community-based organizations can begin to help by recognizing the significant effect the epidemic has on the women who are caring for family members and friends with HIV disease in their personal lives, as well as those who work within the health and social service delivery systems. Supportive programs might include informal rap groups for caretakers, special events recognizing and honoring women who care for people with HIV disease, stress-reduction programs for caretakers, burnout prevention activities, and support groups on grieving or death and dying. The activities listed in Chapter Three include several events that can be planned for caregivers.

Parental Concerns

Talking to children

Not surprisingly, many women are concerned about the health risks their children face during this epidemic. At a series of trainings conducted by the Women's Centers and AIDS Project over a two-year period, one issue was repeatedly raised by attendees: women's concern for their children and anxiety about talking to them about sex, drugs, and HIV. As the primary communicators of sexual and reproductive information to children, women, in particular, need accurate, age-appropriate information for their children, and skills for discussing HIV with sexually active or drug-experimenting adolescents. Adolescence is a time when young people explore the world and their own identities, and may experiment with drugs and sex. Both of these behaviors put them at risk for infection with HIV. Since about 10% of young people are gay or lesbian and many more experiment sexually with members of the same and opposite sexes, education on HIV and sexuality should be inclusive of issues pertaining to gay and lesbian as well as heterosexual youth. Denying young people accurate and non-biased information on sexuality, drugs, and HIV prevention may increase their risk for acquiring HIV infection. It is important to prevent HIV infection in young people by providing them with information, as well as decision-making, communication, and assertiveness skills. This sometimes means putting aside our own feelings of embarrassment about discussing sexual behavior and drug use with young people for the sake of achieving the primary goal of preventing HIV. For more information on HIV and adolescents, see Chapter Six.

Parents need information about how HIV is and is not transmitted.

Children with AIDS

Some women may need information and support in dealing with children who are already infected or ill. While the vast majority (83%) of children with AIDS were infected during pregnancy, 10% of pediatric AIDS cases were the result of blood transfusions, 5% resulted from the use of blood and blood products for hemophilia and coagulation disorders, and the cause of 2% was undetermined (*HIV/AIDS Surveillance Report*, September 1990). There have also been reported cases of children who have been infected through sexual abuse by an infected adult. All parents who have an infected or sick child — whether or not they themselves are also at risk — may need, along with all the usual support offered to the parents of an ill child, assistance in dealing with the stigma that may be experienced by the child and family. This may mean advocating that a child with HIV infection or disease be allowed to remain in school and participate in regular classroom activities, or providing targeted educational programs to raise awareness and understanding in the community about HIV.

Casual contact

Another issue that concerns many parents is the possibility of transmitting HIV through casual contact. HIV *cannot* be transmitted by kissing, hugging, changing diapers, sharing forks and spoons, or through other kinds of daily contact between parents and children. The myth that HIV can be transmitted casually detracts from effective education and prevention, as well as leading to discrimination against and fear of people with HIV disease. Parents need information about how HIV is and is not transmitted. They need to know that it is safe for their children to be in school with children who have HIV infection or disease, and to have contact with adults perceived to be at risk. Finally, all of us — women and men alike — need support in coping with irrational fears about having casual contact with people with HIV disease. These fears are natural, but they must be overcome. As a service provider, you are in an excellent position not only to offer information, but to help people deal with the feelings that this issue will inevitably raise, so that they can get beyond them. This will probably include working with your staff as well as with clients, and providing ongoing reinforcement of accurate messages about how HIV is and is not transmitted.

6

Working with Different Groups of Women

How HIV affects different groups of women

HIV disease impacts women differently, depending upon their social and economic circumstances, the area they live in, the strength of their support systems, their age, the nature of their risk behaviors, the availability of services in their community, and a host of other factors. For this reason, the nature of the prevention information they receive and the degree to which they are reached with services and information, varies. Many groups of women are not included in efforts to reach women with risk-reduction information. Examples of groups that are largely ignored in prevention efforts are older women, disabled women, incarcerated women, and lesbians. Other groups, such as women who work in the sex industry and adolescents, may be the focus of prevention efforts, but too often in ways that are disempowering. Prostitutes are frequently the focus of punitive prevention efforts that seek to punish them rather than to promote their health and safety. They are seen as vectors of transmission to heterosexual men and by extension, to families, rather than as individuals at risk. Adolescents, on the other hand, are often reached with simplistic HIV and drug prevention campaigns that instruct them to "just say no," rather than providing accurate, explicit information and the skills to act on this information. Knowing some of these populations' special issues, women's centers and other CBOs can provide them with appropriate HIV-related information and support. Appendix A lists educational materials that are specifically designed for many of the groups discussed below.

> **Many groups are not included in efforts to reach women with risk-reduction information.**

Adolescents

In recent years, adolescents have become one of the prime targets of HIV prevention information. Because adolescence is a time of exploration and experimentation with sexuality and drug use, there is ample reason to believe that this already affected population will be impacted further by HIV in the years to come. High rates of teen pregnancy, sexually transmitted disease, and drug experimentation and addiction are all indicators that many young people are involved in behaviors that place them at risk.

As of January 1991, a total of 646 cases of AIDS among persons 13-19 years of age had been reported to the Centers for Disease Control (*HIV/AIDS Surveillance Report*, February 1991). Of these cases, 42% are white, 37% are African American, 18% are Latino, and 2% are Asian/Pacific Islanders or Native American/Alaskan Natives. However, looking only at the number of teens who currently have AIDS understates the problem of adolescent infection. The virus' long incubation period means that many of the almost

33,000 adults with AIDS between the ages of 20 and 29 reported to the CDC probably became infected sometime during their teenage years.

Patterns of transmission among adolescents have differed from those of adults in two important ways. The first is that for teens of both sexes, the primary mode of HIV transmission is sex with an infected male. Almost half of the cases of AIDS in adolescent females in the U.S. are the result of heterosexual transmission, as compared with adult women, for whom sex with infected males accounts for approximately one-third of AIDS cases.

The second difference is that the sharing of intravenous drug equipment — the leading risk factor for adult women — is not the primary transmission mode for adolescents, although it accounts for about one-fifth of the AIDS cases among teenage women nationally and almost one-third of New York City's cases among female teens. Intravenous drug use is not prevalent among adolescents; however, substance abuse in its many forms *does* impact significantly the spread of HIV among young persons. The cocaine/crack epidemic among inner-city youth (which is associated with the exchange of sex for money and drugs, heightened sex drive, and disinhibition), drug and alcohol experimentation and addiction among young people (leading to impaired judgment, which hinders the ability and desire to practice sexual risk reduction), and the fact that by the age of eighteen well over half of all American adolescents have become sexually active — all are signals that urgently call for the creation of youth-focused HIV prevention efforts that emphasize both sexual risk reduction and substance abuse prevention and treatment.

Childhood and adolescence are the time when a young person develops his or her attitudes toward sex and sexual decision-making. A comprehensive approach to developing a healthy attitude toward sex and sexual responsibility should include but go beyond an understanding of biological and fact-based information about the reproductive system, disease prevention, and birth control. Young people need to be empowered to make responsible decisions about sex, to change or modify risky behaviors, and should be provided with opportunities to talk about their feelings and concerns about sexual issues and to learn and practice the skills of communication, negotiation, and decision-making. Studies conducted in this country in the past year show that American teens as well as adults are often ignorant of even the most basic and important sexual and reproductive issues — they are "sexually illiterate." The price of failing to educate our children properly about sexual issues has always been high — teenage pregnancy and sexually-transmitted diseases among teens are widespread and increasing in the United States. But now, with HIV, the results of these failings are even more tragic, and the responsibility to educate and support youth in protecting themselves has grown even more important.

As with other groups, many barriers exist to reaching young people with HIV/AIDS prevention information. Beyond the barriers of cultural, religious, and language differences that also exist for adults, there is the taboo of teen sex and the controversy about speaking openly about sexual matters to young people. Meaningful prevention programs for youth must cover not only how to "say no," but what the thousands of American kids who have already "said yes" need to know about sexual health and sexual responsibility. It means helping young people to understand that the HIV epidemic does not mean that sex is a "bad" thing nor that sex equals death; in other words, fostering a healthy approach to sexuality within the context of an epidemic. It also means giving young people factual and understandable information about alcohol and other drugs, and how these substances can impair intelligent sexual decision-making and the exercise of choice. Information of this kind can come from a variety of sources, including parents, the schools, peers, the mass media, and service organizations that come into contact with young people.

Teenagers are not seeing their peers die at the same rate that they are being infected.

When working with adolescents — or any other population — it is important to remember that some of them will be gay or lesbian, and that your information should be designed accordingly. Adolescence is a time when many young people are forming their sexual identities and may experiment sexually with partners of both sexes, even if they consider themselves heterosexual. Others will openly identify as gay or lesbian. Still others will be "closeted." All need to understand that the risk of HIV infection comes from certain unprotected sexual activities, not sexual identity per se. We want to protect all our young people from infection with HIV. Therefore, risk-reduction information should include accurate, non-judgmental information about sexual behavior that is relevant to all.

Another "barrier" issue to be aware of is the perception commonly held by young people that they are impervious to harm. A sense of invulnerability is a normal, age-appropriate perception for teenagers. However, it poses a challenge to service providers who wish to motivate them to protect themselves from HIV, a seemingly vague and distant danger. The virus' long incubation period before the onset of symptoms means that teenagers are not seeing their peers die at the same rate that they are being infected, and thus do not see the risk involved in having unprotected sexual intercourse or using drugs. Helping this present-oriented population make the conceptual leap that what they do this week may harm them in five years is an intrinsic part of doing effective prevention with this group. It is a slow and ongoing process.

If your organization serves young people, it can become involved in HIV/AIDS prevention in a number of ways, including screening videos designed for adolescents and following up with group discussions, setting up peer counseling and peer education programs, and planning youth workshops on communication and assertiveness skills. Your organization can adapt many of the activities in Chapter Three to the specific needs of a younger group. The ability to assert oneself, communicate with a sexual partner, maintain control in sexual situations, and protect one's health are as important for sexually active teenage women as for their adult counterparts. If you work with mixed groups of teens, you can also reach male adolescents with the information, skills, and support for practicing safer sex and sexual responsibility.

There are several important issues to consider when planning education efforts for teenagers. Many existing prevention materials for kids use "scare tactics" to frighten young people away from behaviors that put them at risk. This seems like common sense, but scare tactics have limited value since extreme fear also "turns people off" to prevention messages. Also, such approaches fail to offer alternatives to risk-taking behaviors. If we are going to ask our children to give up sex, drugs, drinking, and other risk-taking behaviors, we must be prepared to replace those things with something else. This means going beyond slogans by helping young people develop identities based upon other values, expand and explore their interests, increase their life options, assert themselves, and bolster their self-respect. Positive male and female role models are very important in this regard. As with adults, an effective HIV prevention strategy for teenagers and children will involve dealing with the whole person.

When working with young men and women, it is important to be aware of the sexual double standards that negatively impact young people of both sexes. The double standard puts the onus on young women to assume responsibility for maintaining chastity and sexual limit-setting, while giving young men the message that their status and self-worth as males hinge on their sexual prowess. This system places both women and men in an untenable bind when it comes to practicing safer sex or sexual abstinence. It sets young women up as "easy" (as opposed to "assertive" or "responsible") if they take the initiative to talk about sex and condom use with their partner, and gives young men the message that discussing sex and being sexually responsible are not "macho" behaviors. Young women and men need permission, encouragement, information, and practical skills to break free of the damaging effect of gender stereotypes upon sexual behavior and sexual negotiation. As service providers, our role is to find new ways to "market" safer sex to young people, as well as to adults, and to make communication, mutual respect, and HIV risk reduction desirable behaviors.

With respect to adolescent drug use and abuse, programs such as yours can work to both *prevent* drug abuse among teens and to provide support to those who are already struggling with drug and alcohol dependence. Prevention efforts should go beyond slogans and abstinence campaigns to address the context in which drug abuse occurs. It may be unavoidable that many young people will experiment with drugs, but the route from experimentation to addiction may be hastened by other factors such as low self-esteem, limited economic, recreational, or social alternatives, and the desire to "escape" from painful or difficult personal circumstances. Effective prevention programs must not occur in a vacuum, but should address these issues, offering young people meaningful alternatives to drug and alcohol abuse and other self-destructive behaviors.

Intervention for young persons who are *already* addicted means becoming sensitive to hidden addictions, and providing addicted teens with direct intervention and referrals to youth-serving treatment programs, support groups, and relapse prevention services. This may also involve advocating that local drug programs provide age-appropriate services to young people in the community.

Even if your center does not work with adolescents, it can have an impact on young people through its work with adults. Your adult clients are the mothers, aunts, and sisters of young people. You can teach them the skills for communicating with young people and each other about HIV, sex, and drugs, and persuade them of the importance of doing so. In doing so, you can make a contribution toward reaching young people through their family network.

Lesbians

Society's heavy reliance on the notion of "risk groups" has rendered lesbians one of the most invisible groups of women with HIV/AIDS, an extension of the larger lack of recognition of lesbians in our culture. The relatively low incidence of HIV infection among lesbians is often taken to mean that women who have sex with women are somehow "magically protected" or immune from HIV infection. Of course, like everybody else, lesbians can and do become infected if they engage in high-risk drug-related and sexual activities. Behavior, not sexual identity, determines an individual's level of risk.

Some lesbians are at risk for HIV infection from having unprotected sex with men, some through sharing IV drug equipment, and others from artificial insemination by an infected donor. Although statistics are not kept on lesbians with AIDS per se, according to the Centers for Disease Control, most lesbians with HIV were infected through the sharing of IV needles and "works."

Provide the full spectrum of safer sex and prevention information to all audiences.

Very little is known (because almost no research has been done) about the risk of sexual transmission of HIV between women. Most cases of woman-to-woman transmission are anecdotal. However, we do know that HIV is found in the blood (including menstrual blood), vaginal secretions, semen, breast milk, and urine of infected persons, so any behaviors that pass these fluids from one person's body into another's are considered risky. Safer sex guidelines for lesbians have been developed based upon what is known about HIV transmission generally. These guidelines form a point of departure for women wishing to consider adopting risk reduction activities. Appendix A contains a listing of lesbian-specific AIDS education materials, some of which include safer sex guidelines for women who have sex with women.

Groups providing risk reduction information and HIV services can insure that lesbians receive the information they need by making lesbian-appropriate information available to the women they serve, regardless of whether lesbians are a recognized part of the caseload or targeted audience. Always assume that there will be a range of sexual orientations represented in your target population, and provide the full spectrum of safer sex and prevention information to all audiences to insure that everyone — lesbian, heterosexual, and bisexual — will leave your program with all the information they need.

Women's centers can promote the idea that invisibility is not the same thing as immunity, and can motivate lesbians to assess their own risk levels and to work toward protecting themselves, their partners, and their communities. Remember that many lesbians will also need support as caretakers of gay male friends with HIV disease. CBOs can provide support to lesbians who are themselves HIV positive, and can offer assistance to their partners and caretakers by creating an environment that addresses their needs. Agencies such as yours can also make sure that other AIDS-funded agencies are inclusive of lesbian issues when developing safer sex materials, providing services, and promoting HIV awareness.

Incarcerated women

Throughout the country, incarcerated women (as well as men) have been disproportionately affected by the HIV epidemic. The proportion of incarcerated women who are at risk for HIV because of their histories of IV drug use is significantly higher than that of the overall population of women. Many other women in prison are at risk from sex with partners who are infected with HIV, usually through the sharing of IV drug paraphernalia. Still others are at risk from having engaged in "survival sex," prostitution for drugs and/or money. In some states, women engaged in prostitution have been incarcerated only because they are HIV-infected.

Despite the soaring rates of HIV disease among incarcerated persons in the United States, prison systems in most states and counties have been largely unresponsive to the crisis. Critical concerns for HIV-positive women in prison include lack of appropriate assistance with substance abuse problems, discrimination, lack of medical confidentiality, abuse by frightened and misinformed prison staff and fellow prisoners, and most importantly, inadequate psychosocial and medical care and lack of access to life-prolonging treatments. For both HIV-positive women and those who are not infected, concerns also include the absence of prevention information and AIDS education.

> **Prison systems in most states have been unresponsive to the crisis.**

Throughout the country, women in prison settings have taken active roles in providing for their own HIV education, supporting each other through illness and the loss of loved ones, fighting discrimination, and advocating for appropriate HIV-related medical and social services. This has happened with help and support from those on the "outside" who believe that everyone is entitled to adequate health care and support in coping with the epidemic. Concerned women's groups and CBOs can play a variety of roles in helping to improve the conditions of incarcerated women who are affected by HIV. They can advocate for AIDS education/training for prisoners as well as the personnel with whom they interact daily. They can act as "watchdogs" on prison conditions and press for more appropriate medical and social services for those who need them. They can provide support for HIV positive as well as uninfected women upon or prior to their release from prison. They can develop AIDS education materials that are appropriate for women in the prison setting, or offer to donate existing materials to the women inside. And they can provide safer sex workshops, educational and empowerment programs, and technical assistance to groups wishing to initiate their own HIV-related activities and support systems.

Older women

Stereotypes concerning older adults, especially women, represent them as asexual. This myth, combined with the overall invisibility of older women in our society and a general lack of attention to their health-related needs, means that they fall low on the list of groups to be reached with HIV-related information. The fact is that while women of childbearing age have been and will continue to be hardest hit, there are older women (and men) who have HIV infection and illness. Since most women are sexually active throughout their adult lives, HIV prevention information should be provided across the board, regardless of age. CBOs that serve women of various ages can help by giving HIV-related information to all their clients, and not assuming that older women do not need this information. They can also help by encouraging sexually active older women to indentify their own special concerns — whether they be related to sexual communication, using condoms again after years of not needing birth control, or other issues.

Older women who are not themselves at risk will often have the same HIV-related concerns as their younger counterparts if their family members, friends, or work colleagues are confronting HIV in their personal and/or professional lives. Those caring for family members with HIV disease will need information about support services for themselves and their families and may have fears about casual contact and transmission. As aunts, mothers, grandmothers, and friends, older women are often conduits of important reproductive and health-related knowledge to younger women. If properly educated, they can play an important role in passing along important HIV-related information to others. They may also be able to draw on their past experiences to lend insight on issues of bereavement and death to those who are experiencing the loss of friends and family from HIV disease.

Women who are physically challenged

In many of the same ways that older women are often invisible in the eyes of the larger culture, so too are the physically challenged. Disabled women are also frequently presumed to be asexual and are thus overlooked by many programs doing AIDS outreach, creating educational materials, or disseminating information. When your center serves women with disabilities, it is important to make appropriate information available to them on the same range of issues you provide for your other clients. Ideally, that would mean finding materials for women who are blind, hearing impaired, or have some other physical disability. However, few such materials exist at present, so organizations wishing to reach physically disabled women may need to respond to the lack of materials by creating their own, or working with their local AIDS organization to see that educational media that are appropriate for these groups are developed.

Just as there are a variety of different disabilities which affect people, there are different issues to consider when offering AIDS education and services to these populations. If one is working with a population with mobility impairments, access will be a priority — are the meeting rooms wheelchair accessible by ramps and/or elevators? If your center wishes to offer HIV prevention information to women who are visually impaired, the media used to convey this information must be in braille, on audio cassette, or in large print. The Surgeon General's AIDS education booklet is available in braille as are other prevention materials. See Appendix A for more information about HIV resources for the blind or visually impaired and the hearing impaired.

Special issues for female sex workers

Many women's centers have had contact with sex workers — street prostitutes, call girls, escorts, and women who sometimes supplement their income by selling sex or who exchange sex for drugs. In the early days of the AIDS epidemic, sex workers were one of the supposed "high risk groups" and were blamed for the virus' spread into the "general population." In fact, research has shown that prostitutes have a lower infection rate than was previously assumed, and that most of those infected had shared infected IV drug equipment. Although these findings have helped to reduce the undue focus on prostitutes who practice their trade, sex workers bear the brunt of a legally enforced double standard in which their male clients are perceived as in need of special protection while they are viewed as perpetrating "crimes."

Some agencies will wish to help such women to protect themselves against HIV infection by offering them prevention information and access to condoms and other safer sex materials. Many sex workers already use condoms and insist on having safer sex. Others do not. Depending on a woman's access to health information, her economic status, and the conditions under which she works, the practice of safer sex may be more or less difficult for her to manage. For example, a woman who works as a highly paid call girl in settings where health rules are followed will have an easier time practicing risk reduction (and protecting her safety in other respects) than someone who is working on the streets without external support, protection, or control over the circumstances under which she must operate.

Women who have developed safer sex techniques while "on the job" may be ideal role models and teachers for other sex workers seeking to integrate this form of self-protection into their paid work. As with any group of women, HIV prevention and safer sex education should occur within the larger context of empowerment, self-esteem, and health promotion. Your program may be able to help (directly or through referral) sex workers who do not have access to general health care, drug treatment, psychosocial services, and support for practicing safer sex. For many, the first step to self-protection will be coping with IV drug use or other addicitons — the primary route of transmission for HIV-positive sex workers (and women generally) and a serious impediment to the clear judgment required for insisting upon safer sex.

Other issues you may want to consider are:

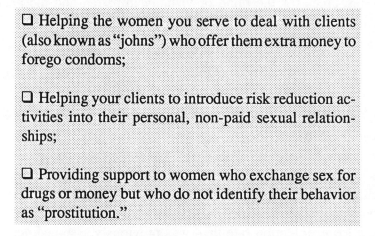

❑ Helping the women you serve to deal with clients (also known as "johns") who offer them extra money to forego condoms;

❑ Helping your clients to introduce risk reduction activities into their personal, non-paid sexual relationships;

❑ Providing support to women who exchange sex for drugs or money but who do not identify their behavior as "prostitution."

Your agency may already provide services to sex workers, or serve clients who participate in these activities but do not self-identify as such. By exhibiting an awareness of these issues and sensitivity to the social and economic realities that lead women to either select or resort to sex work, you can help to support an underserved population for whom safer sex is especially complicated. See Appendix A for a listing of HIV education materials designed for women in the sex industry.

Conclusion

*W*omen, AIDS, & Communities: A Guide for Action has attempted to provide a basic understanding of key HIV/AIDS issues, with an emphasis on those with particular relevance to women. It has described some of the special ways that the epidemic impacts specific groups, and has suggested possible activities for organizations like yours to take on, along with an overview of the resources available to help you.

Most importantly, however, this guide has provided a rationale for the involvement of grass roots or community-based organizations in providing gender-specific HIV information, education, skills, and direct services for women. We hope that as the HIV-related "gaps" in your community become apparent, you will consider applying some of your organization's skills and energies toward filling them.

As with most social and health-related movements, the first (and many of the best) responses to AIDS were born of community action and were based upon an understanding of and respect for the populations for whom they were created. Most often, they were created by those most heavily impacted by the epidemic. As the range of communities affected continues to grow, so does the diversity of responses being initiated.

The rapid growth in the number of women with HIV disease in the U.S. has meant that the past few years have seen the development of more women-focused programs. However, grass roots activity on women and AIDS issues must become much more widespread in order to reach the ever-increasing numbers of women and families affected by the health emergency. This will only happen through the interest and initiative of affected communities and their allies, with support from existing groups.

The HIV/AIDS epidemic has been with us for ten years. In that time, the "AIDS field" has become increasingly "professionalized." Too often, the role of community, informal, or non-institutional involvement in confronting the crisis is overlooked, under-recognized, and underfunded. This "professionalization" has sometimes discouraged the involvement of AIDS "newcomers." It is our view that community involvement is crucial to the success of both HIV prevention and service programs, and that it represents a vital counterpoint to more centralized and institutional forms of HIV prevention and care that have developed over the past decade. A diversity of approaches is crucial to maintaining a vital and strong HIV/AIDS prevention and service effort.

It is our hope that the creativity and energy of the grassroots approach from which this movement was born will not get lost in the shuffle of a developing "AIDS bureaucracy," nor be diminished by the

Grass roots activity on women and AIDS issues must become much more widespread.

growing struggle over a limited funding and resources pie. If nothing else, as organizations and individuals, we can advocate strongly for increases in the amount of financial and technical resources allotted to this particular issue so that constructive action can be maintained and expanded at all levels.

In discussing the role of CBOs in this guide, we have focused on two main issues: HIV education/prevention and direct services (including health and social services). With regard to prevention, it is widely recognized that health messages are most likely to be accepted when the source of these messages is perceived as trustworthy. Such credibility is based on whether the source is seen as recognizing and reflecting the individual or community's point of view and values — in other words, whether or not it is a "friend" of the community. This is especially important when, as is the case with HIV/AIDS, the messages are controversial, frightening, or involve taboo subjects like sex and drugs.

An organization that has already won a community's trust is well-situated to deliver effective health-promoting messages. And it can also do something which is even more important: foster an environment where the behavioral changes needed for HIV prevention are encouraged and ultimately normalized. A group that is truly responsive to its constituency will know best how to promote such changes within the context of its community's needs, realities, and attitudes.

The same holds true for delivering direct services for people with HIV disease, their caretakers, and their loved ones. A group that knows its community well can provide the most appropriate and "user friendly" services, given the proper resources to do so. Direct services can be tailored to suit the needs of those being served vis-à-vis such factors as hours, location, language(s) spoken, types of services offered and the style in which they are delivered. Groups with an understanding of women's issues will be able to apply their knowledge to developing gender-appropriate services for women at risk and those already affected by HIV. They can also make sure that other HIV programs are accessible to women, and that women are not "forgotten" when HIV-related policies, funding, and activities are initiated.

For all of these reasons, we want to encourage you to become active, whether on a large or small scale, in addressing some of the many existing and emerging issues of women and AIDS — from HIV prevention to direct services, from AIDS activism to advocacy — in both urban and rural areas. We hope that this guidebook will provide some impetus for doing so.

Appendices

EDUCATIONAL MATERIALS

There is a wide array of materials intended to educate people about HIV/AIDS. Some of these are targeted to women and communities of color. Booklets, pamphlets, posters, fliers, videotapes, and newsletters can be effective in training staff, doing advocacy, educating clients, and generally increasing the visibility of the HIV issue in your organization.

The Women's Centers and AIDS Project has produced "A Guide To Educational Materials" which lists AIDS education materials that are geared to women. The complete 16-page listing is available for $2.25 from WCAP, c/o Women's Action Alliance, 370 Lexington Avenue, Suite 603, New York, NY 10017. Below is an updated and abbreviated listing of materials which may be useful in your work.

"Acquired Immune Deficiency Syndrome and Victims of Sexual Violence" (policy paper). Pennsylvania Coalition Against Rape's (PCAR) Policy Issue Paper #3. Prepared by Barbara A. Nissley and Susan J. Cameron. Designed for those working with victims of sexual violence, this paper contains current information on victims, offenders, and HIV infection and AIDS. Order from: PCAR, 2300 North Third Street, Harrisburg, PA 17110, (717) 232-6745. Price: $10.

"AIDS and Deafness Directory." Available from the National AIDS Information Clearinghouse, (800) 458-5231, order #B-070.

"AIDS and Domestic Violence" (fact sheet). Discusses the often tenuous position battered women are in concerning HIV/AIDS prevention and safer sex negotiation. Suggests methods service providers can use to effectively counsel them. One page. Order from: Connecticut Coalition Against Domestic Violence, (203) 524-5890.

"AIDS and Prostitution." AIDS Prevention Among Female Sexual Partners of Intravenous Drug Users Annotated Bibliography. Order from: NOVA Research, (301) 986-1891.

"AIDS and Vision Loss Conference Proceedings" (sound recordings). Produced by the Lighthouse, American Foundation for the Blind, January 1990. Available from: Conference Audio Services (San Francisco, CA), (415) 775-8273.

"AIDS Antibody Testing at Alternative Test Sites" (booklet). Provides information to help make an informed decision about whether or not to take the HIV antibody test. Although written for the San Francisco area, it is informative for anyone considering the test. This and related information are available from the San Francisco AIDS Foundation, 333 Valencia Street, P.O. Box 6182, San Francisco, CA 94101-6182, (415) 861-3397.

"AIDS Discrimination Posters." Available free of charge from the New York City Commission on Human Rights. Three attractive posters, each loosely geared to a different population: "Diana and the Supremes," African-American (English and Spanish); "Baseball," Latino (English and Spanish); and "Woodstock," white (English only). To order, call (212) 566-8974, or write to the Commission at: 52 Duane Street, New York, NY 10007.

"AIDS, HIV and Domestic Violence" (paper). A discussion piece for supervisors. Provides support, training, and supervision to battered women's counselors and advocates. How counselors can work with battered women on issues of AIDS, rape, sexuality, infidelity, drug abuse, and other topics which are often difficult to discuss. 20 pages. February 1990. Available from: Connecticut Coalition Against Domestic Violence, (203) 524-5890. Price: cost of postage.

"AIDS in the Black Community" (booklet). Produced by the New York Urban League. Discusses issues for Black gay men, IV drug users, women, and children, as well as discrimination and the epidemic's impact on the community as a whole. Order from: New York Urban League, 218 West 40th Street, New York, NY 10018, (212) 730-5200.

"AIDS: Information About the Ethical, Medical and Legal Issues Relevant to Policy Development for Domestic Violence Programs" (policy paper). Connecticut Coalition Against Domestic Violence developed this paper for counselors serving battered women. 1988. Order from: Connecticut Coalition Against Domestic Violence, (203) 524-5890. Price: cost of postage (approximately $7).

"AIDS Information Resources Directory." A Review of over 400 pamphlets, videotapes, curricula, posters, and books. Order from: R.R. Bowker, 245 West 17th Street, New York, NY 10011. In New York City, call (212) 337-6934. Outside New York City, call (800) 521-8110.

"AIDS Is About Secrets" (video). An empowering video geared to Black women whose partners are IV drug users; the issues it raises will resonate with other audiences as well. The same producer has also made a video called "AIDS: Not Us," which is targeted to young inner city men and supports male responsibility for safer sex. Both videos are credible and engaging. For preview, rental, and purchase information contact: The Film Library, Claire Walsh and Associates, 22 Florida Avenue, Staten Island, NY 10305, (718)720-4488.

"AIDS Legal Guide." Written by Abby R. Rubenfeld for legal professionals on the legal problems of AIDS. Order from: LAMBDA Legal Defense and Education Fund, Inc., 666 Broadway, New York, NY 10012, (212) 995-8585.

"AIDS Prevention and Education: Reframing the Message." A synthesis of current research and understanding on policy issues related to HIV prevention and education programs. Available free of charge from: Citizens' Commission on AIDS, 121 Avenue of the Americas, 6th Floor, New York, NY 10013, (212)925-5290.

"AIDS Service Directory for Hispanics." Order from: COSSMHO, 1030 15th Street, NW, Suite 1053, Washington, DC 20005, (202) 371-2100. Price: $7.50.

AIDS: The Women (book). Edited by Ines Rieder and Patricia Ruppelt. A collection of writings by women on AIDS. Order from: Cleis East, P.O. Box 8933, Pittsburgh, PA 15221, or Cleis West, P.O. Box 14684, San Francisco, CA 94114. Paperback price: $9.95 plus $1.50 shipping (PA and CA residents add sales tax).

AIDS Treatment News (biweekly newsletter). Contains reports on experimental and alternative treatments, information from medical journals, and more. Order from: ATN Publications, P.O. Box 411256, San Francisco, CA 94141, (415) 255-0588. Price: $100 per year ($30 for persons with AIDS or ARC or HIV infection; $150 for organizations).

"AIDS: What the Deaf Should Know" (brochure). Available from AIDS Education for the Deaf, 8350 Santa Monica Blvd., West Hollywood, CA 90069, or call (213) 654-5942; TDD: (213) 654-5822.

American Bar Association Immigration Law Implementation Project offers a packet of materials for persons applying for amnesty or practitioners counseling seropositive immigrants. Order from: American Immigration Lawyers Association, 1000 16th Street, NW, Suite 604, Washington, DC 20036, Attention: Legalization Issues Bank. Specify Document # L0488-153. Contact person: Carol Wolchok, (202) 331-2268. Price: $17.

American College Health Association (ACHA) offers AIDS pamphlets for college students covering safer sex, sexual decision-making, women and AIDS, and more. Order from: ACHA, 1300 Piccard Drive, Suite 200, Rockville, MD 20855, (301) 963-1100.

"Annotated Bibliography on Women and AIDS." Prepared by NOVA Research Company in conjunction with NIDA's National AIDS Demonstration Research (NADR) Project. Order from: National Clearinghouse on Alcohol and Drug Information, P.O. Box 2345, Rockville, MD 20852. Order number RP0728. Comprehensive Bibliography.

Body Positive (monthly holistic/alternative newsletter). Letters, articles, and announcements on the medical, social, and psychological concerns of HIV-positive people. Order from: Body Positive, 2095 Broadway, Suite 306, New York, NY 10023, (212) 721-1346. Subscription: $25 per year.

Center for Population Options offers educational materials targeting teens aged 12-19. HIV issues are covered in fact sheets, bibliographies, and conference reports. For information, contact: CPO, Publications department, 1012 14th Street, NW, Room 1200, Washington, DC 20005, (202) 347-5700.

"The Child with AIDS: A Guide for the Family." Order from: AIDS Program, Children's Hospital of New Jersey, 15 South 9th Street, Newark, NJ 07107, (201) 268-8273.

Chinatown Health Clinic - AIDS Project offers pamphlets in Chinese covering various HIV issues including those for women and children. Order from: Chinatown Health Clinic - AIDS Project, Health Education Department, 89 Baxter Street, New York, NY 10013, (212) 732-9547.

COSSMHO AIDS Update (monthly newsletter). Focuses on the Latino community, covering issues from fundraising to Latino newsmakers in the AIDS field. Order from: COSSMHO, 1030 15th Street, NW, Suite 1053, Washington, DC 20005, (202) 371-2100. Price: $40 ($30 for members).

The Exchange (newsletter). Discusses issues of concern to service providers working with survivors of domestic violence. The Fall/Winter 1988-89 Vol. 3, No. 1. issue includes "Responding to the AIDS Crisis: The Challenge to Shelters." Order from: National Woman Abuse Prevention Project, 2000 P Street, N.W., Suite 508, Washington, DC 20036.

Haitian Coalition on AIDS. Printed materials in Creole and English available on teens, children, adults and HIV, transmission, etc. Contact the Haitian Centers Council, Inc., Haitian Coalition on AIDS, 50 Court Street, Suite 605, Brooklyn, NY 11201, (718) 855-7275/6.

"Hard to Get" (video). Narrated by Ruby Dee, is an entertaining training video about AIDS discrimination in the work place. Available free to AIDS trainers and others. 18 minutes. To order, call the New York City Commission on Human Rights at (212) 566-5177 or write to the Commission at: 52 Duane Street, New York, NY 10007.

HIV/AIDS Surveillance Report. Published each month by the Division of HIV/AIDS, Center for Infectious Diseases, Centers for Disease Control. An expanded, year-end edition is published each January. Copies are available free from the National AIDS Information Clearinghouse, P.O. Box 6003, Rockville, MD 20850. Individuals or organizations can be added to the mailing list by contacting the Centers for Disease Control, Division of HIV/AIDS, Technical Information Activity, Mailstop G-29, Atlanta, GA 30333.

"HIV-Related Discrimination by Reproductive Health Care Providers in New York City" (report). Available free from the New York City Commission on Human Rights, (212) 566-8974 or write to the Commission at: 52 Duane Street, New York, NY 10007.

"It's Not Just Hearing AIDS: Deaf People and the Epidemic" (videotape/film). For ordering/cost information write: Deaf AIDS Project, 1046 North Martel Street, West Hollywood, CA 90046.

"Learning AIDS: An Information Resource Directory." Produced by AmFar (American Foundation for AIDS Research). Order from R.R. Bowker at (800) 521-8110. In New York, call (212) 337-6934. Price: $24.95.

"Lesbians and AIDS: What's the Connection?" (brochure). Addresses safer sex, transmission, risk factors, and the emotional and political impact of AIDS upon the lesbian community. Order from: San Francisco AIDS Foundation, 333 Valencia Street, P.O. Box 6182, San Francisco, CA 94101-6182, (415) 861-3397.

"Living with AIDS" (signed/captioned video for the hearing impaired). Available from Gallaudet University, Merrill Learning Center, Department of Television, Film, and Photography, 800 Florida Avenue, NE, Room LN30, Washington, DC 20002, (202) 651-5115. Ask for video #312.

"Living with AIDS: A Guide to the Legal Problems of People with AIDS" (booklet) includes: accessing services, protecting confidentiality, insurance issues, and more. Order from: LAMBDA Legal Defense and Education Fund, Inc., 666 Broadway, New York, NY 10012, (212) 995-8585.

Making It: A Woman's Guide to Sex in the Age of AIDS (book). Written in English by Cindy Patton and Janis Kelly, and translated into Spanish by Papusa Molina, this work covers most issues heterosexual, bisexual, and lesbian women face in the age of the AIDS crisis. Includes information on artificial insemination, negotiation, risk assessment, and eroticizing safer sex. Order from: Firebrand Books, 141 The Commons, Ithaca, NY 14850, (607) 272-0000. Purchase price: $3.95 plus $1.50 for shipping. For service organizations, orders of 25 or more are offered at a 60% discount plus shipping costs.

"Masks/Mascaras" (video). Developed by the Hispanic AIDS Forum, this video targets Latinas who are intravenous drug users or sexual partners of IV drug users. It is intended for use by social service organizations that are not AIDS-focused. For more information, contact: Hispanic AIDS Forum at (212) 966-6336.

"Me First! Medical Manifestations of HIV in Women" (brochure). Describes the problem of under-diagnosis of HIV in women and the gynecological symptoms many HIV positive women manifest. Discusses a variety of female-specific health issues related to HIV, including pelvic inflammatory disease, chancroid, candida, HPV and neoplasia, syphilis, and herpes simplex virus. Available from: the New Jersey Women and AIDS Network (NJWAN), 5 Elm Row, New Brunswick, NJ 08901.

"Medical Answers About AIDS" (booklet). Published by the Gay Men's Health Crisis (GMHC), this handbook answers common medical questions. This and many other materials (including a brochure geared to women and one for lesbians) can be ordered from: GMHC 129 West 20th Street, New York, NY 10011, (212) 807-7517.

Narcotic and Drug Research, Inc., Training Institute provides materials on women, substance abuse, and HIV. In both English and Spanish, topics covered include: women and sexual relations with bisexual men and IV drug users, women as IV drug users, and pregnancy and AIDS. Order from: NDRI, Training Institute, 11-17 Beach Street, New York, NY 10013, (212) 966-8700. Price: Free.

The National Native American AIDS Prevention Center. A network of Native American AIDS activists assisting local Native American communities and health groups with information, materials, and training. For more information contact the Center at: 6239 College Avenue, Suite 201, Oakland, CA 94618, (415) 658-2051.

"National Prison Project Annual Statistical Survey of AIDS in Prison and Booklet for Prisoners and Staff." Order from: Judy Greenspan, 1616 P Street, NW, Washington, DC, 20036, (202) 331-0500.

"The New Tradition: Safer Sex Counseling in Family Planning Clinics" (video). Released by Planned Parenthood of Bergen County, this video helps family planning and health agencies integrate AIDS education into their regular activities. 1988: 30 minutes. Part of a package that includes staff training materials, pamphlets, a condom sampler, and more. Order from: Planned Parenthood of Bergen County, 575 Main Street, Hackensack, NJ 07601, (201) 489-1265. Purchase price: $89 plus $3 for postage and handling.

New York Minority AIDS Task Force offers materials on a variety of AIDS issues in English, Spanish, Chinese, and Creole. Order from: NY Minority AIDS Task Force, 92 Saint Nicholas Avenue, Apt. 1B, New York, NY 10026, (212) 749-2816.

New York State Women and AIDS Project Newsletter includes nationwide resources, upcoming conferences, and updates on women and AIDS. Order from: Lynne McArthur, New York State Division of Alcoholism and Alcohol Abuse, Women and AIDS Project, 194 Washington Avenue, Albany, NY 12210.

People With AIDS Coalition publishes a monthly newsletter which consists of current AIDS-related events and issues, personal accounts, local services, support group listings, medical updates, and treatment information. Free to low-income PWAs, $35.00 to others. Contact: PWA Coalition, 31 West 26th Street, 5th Floor, New York, NY 10010, (212) 532-0290.

Preventing AIDS: A Guide to Effective Education for the Prevention of HIV Infection (book). Written by Nicholas Freudenberg, this book discusses how to plan AIDS prevention programs and educate populations such as intravenous drug users, women, prisoners, homeless people, and people with developmental disabilities. Available for $28.50 from: the American Public Health Association, 1015 Fifteenth Street, N.W., Suite 300, Washington, DC 20005, (202) 789-5600.

"Prostitutes Prevent AIDS: A Manual for Health Educators." Written by Priscilla Alexander for organizations who want to implement AIDS prevention programs to help prostitutes protect themselves and others from HIV infection. Order from: CAL-PEP, 333 Valencia Street, Suite 213, San Francisco, CA 94193, (415) 558-0450. Price: $25 plus $2 for shipping.

"Protection Against Infection for Women Using Alternative Insemination" (booklet). This nine-page booklet includes information on protection against infection with HIV and STDs for women using alternative insemination. Order from: The Feminist Institute Clearinghouse, P.O. Box 30563, Bethesda, MD 20814, (301) 951-9040. Price: $4.00.

"Rape, Sexual Assault, and AIDS" (fact sheet). Offers information on what types of sexual assault put a survivor at greater risk of HIV infection. Order from: San Francisco Department of Public Health, Sexual Transmission Services, 50 Ivy Street, San Francisco, CA 94102, (415) 558-3824.

"Rape Victims' Concerns about Possible Exposure to HIV Infection" (research report by T. Baker, et al.). Printed in the *Journal of Interpersonal Violence*, 5(1), 49-60. March 1990. Order from: Victim Services Agency, Research Department, 2 Lafayette Street, New York, NY 10007 (212) 577-7700.

"Responding to AIDS: Ten Principles for the Workplace." Guidelines for a policy on AIDS in the workplace. Order from: Citizens' Commission on AIDS for New York City and Northern New Jersey, 12 Avenue of the Americas, 6th Floor, New York, NY 10013, (212) 925-5290. Price: Free.

"Safer Sex Shorts" (video). A series of brief, explicit safer sex scenarios, all but one intended for gay male audiences. The other "short" is a lesbian safer sex scene depicting the use of dental dams and other risk reduction techniques. In addition, GMHC distributes a brochure entitled "Women Need to Know About AIDS," and has recently developed a new brochure on lesbians and AIDS called "Women Loving Women: Safer Sex." Available from: Gay Men's Health Crisis, 129 West 20th Street, New York, NY 10011-0022, (212)337-3697.

"Se Met Ko" (video). provides HIV information in Haitian Creole with English subtitles. Available from the Haitian Women's Program of the American Friends Service Committee, 15 Rutherford Place, New York, NY 10003, (212)598-0966. Rental fee is $35.00; also available for purchase.

"Seeing Through AIDS" (catalog). A guide to over 70 high-quality AIDS-related films and videos, including many focusing on the politics of AIDS, racial/ethnic minorities, and women. Order from: Media Network, 121 Fulton Street, 5th Floor, New York, NY 10038, (212)619-3455. Price for individuals and low-budget organizations: $6.50 plus $2.00 shipping/handling.

"We Care: A Video for Care Providers of People Affected by AIDS" (video). Developed by the Women's AIDS Video Enterprise, a "video support group" sponsored by the Brooklyn AIDS Task Force and arts funding organizations. For six months, seven women of diverse backgrounds met to learn about AIDS and video. This 32-minute video is the group's final project. Available for $30.00 from: Brooklyn AIDS Task Force, 22 Chapel Street, Brooklyn, NY 11201 (contact: Glenda Smith).

"A Woman's Guide to AIDS" (booklet). Contains basic HIV/AIDS information, safer sex guidelines for heterosexual and lesbian women, and information on pregnancy, children, and care giving. Includes resources for women in the New York City area. Free of charge. To request an order form, call the New York City Department of Health, Office of Public Health Education, (212) 566-8170.

Women, AIDS, and Activism (book). By ACT UP NY (AIDS Coalition to Unleash Power). Women and AIDS Book Group. Spanish edition forthcoming in 1991. South End Press, 300 Raritan Center Parkway, P.O. Box 7816, Edison, NJ 08818-7816. $7.00; free to women in prison.

Women and AIDS (book) by Diane Richardson. Covers the social and psychological impact of AIDS on women. Order from: Methuen Inc., 29 West 35th Street, New York, NY 10001, (212) 244-3336. Paperback price: $9.95.

"Women and AIDS: The Silent Epidemic" (booklet). Provides an overview of the impact of the AIDS crisis on women. Published by the Women's AIDS Resource Network, P.O. Box 020525, 55 Johnson Street, Suite 303, General Building, Brooklyn, NY 11202, (718)596-6008. Free of charge.

Women's AIDS Network provides support, information, technical assistance, and materials on women and AIDS to its members. It has produced an information packet on women and AIDS ($10.00, free to women with HIV) and publishes monthly meeting minutes and announcements. Annual membership is $20.00 for individuals, $50.00 for institutions, $7.50 for low-income individuals, and free to women with HIV. Contact: Women's AIDS Network, c/o San Francisco AIDS Foundation, P.O. Box 6182, San Francisco, CA 94101-6182 or call (415) 864-4376 x2007.

The Young Adult Institute (YAI) has developed a program for sexually active developmentally disabled adults on AIDS education and prevention. Contact: Raymond Jacobs, YAI, 460 West 34th Street, 11th Floor, New York, NY 10001, (212) 563-7474.

B

SERVICE ORGANIZATIONS

Knowing about service organizations in your area is an important part of networking and gaining support as you begin to plan and implement your new HIV activities. The following is a selection from the Women's Centers and AIDS Project's (WCAP) lists of key organizations and service providers in New York and New Jersey, as well as nationally. For a copy of the full 14-page listings of New York Services or New Jersey Services (both of which include a few national groups), send $2.50 per list to the Women's Action Alliance, 370 Lexington Avenue, Suite 603, New York, NY 10017.

Please note: Many of the organizations listed under New York State and New Jersey also provide information, resource materials, referrals, and technical assistance to individuals and agencies throughout the United States.

NEW YORK STATE

AIDS Institute
Empire State Plaza
Corning Tower, Room 359
Albany, NY 12237
Office: (518) 473-7238
Hotline: (800) 541-2437

• Provides regional AIDS coordination and hotlines.

American Friends Service Committee
Haitian Women's Program
New York Metropolitan Region
15 Rutherford Place
New York, NY 10003
Office: (212) 598-0965 (contact Patricia Benoit)

• Offers community education and outreach in Creole and French.

Caribbean Women's Health Association
2725 Church Avenue
Brooklyn, NY 11226
Office: (718) 826-2942

• Provides: community outreach, individual counseling, support groups for HIV-positive persons and their families, information, and referrals. Creole, French, and Spanish are spoken.

Gay Men's Health Crisis
129 West 20th Street
New York, NY 10011
Office: (212) 807-6664
Hotline: (212) 807-6655

• Services provided include: case management, buddy programs, counseling, education, publications, home healthcare workers, referrals, support groups (including those for mothers of children with AIDS), and speakers bureau. Spanish is spoken.

The Hetrick-Martin Institute
401 West Street
New York, NY 10014
Office: (212) 633-8920
TTY for the deaf: (212) 633-8926

• Services for gay, lesbian, and HIV-positive youth: HIV/AIDS counseling, safer sex training, and outreach to the deaf. Also offers training and information to youth-serving professionals.

Hispanic AIDS Forum
121 Avenue of the Americas, Suite 505
New York, NY 10003
(212) 966-6336

• Provides: education, seminars, materials, advocacy, and speakers.

Minority Task Force on AIDS
92 Saint Nicholas Avenue, Apt. 1B
New York, NY 10026
Office: (212) 749-2816
Women's Hotline: (212) 749-3075

• Provides: educational programs, referrals, support groups, speakers, etc.

New York State Division of Human Rights
State Discrimination Unit
55 West 125th Street
New York, NY 10027
Office: (212) 870-8400
24-hr. Hotline for counseling and assistance: (800) 342-AIDS
24-hr. Hotline for testing and counseling: (800) 872-2777

• Provides state-wide referrals to 14 regional offices.

PWA (People With AIDS) Coalition
31 West 26th Street, 5th Floor
New York, NY 10010
Office: (212) 532-0290
Hotline: (212) 532-0568   10 am - 6 pm, Mon-Fri

• Provides: educational programs, referrals, buddy services, support groups, speakers, advocacy, weekly dinners for persons with AIDS, meal delivery for the homebound, and support groups for women with AIDS, ARC, Worried Wells, etc.

Women and AIDS Project
2 World Trade Center, 5th Floor
New York, NY 10047
Office: (212) 587-4408

• Works to bring together organizations which deal with women's concerns around the AIDS epidemic. Offers: education, networking opportunities, occasional newsletter with national relevance, and meetings in New York City, Albany, and Long Island. Contact Annamarie Lewis.

Women and AIDS Resource Network (WARN)
55 Johnson Street
General Building, Suite 303
Brooklyn, NY 11202
Office: (718) 596-6007/8

• Offers counseling, support, advocacy, referrals, workshops, and a speakers bureau.

NEW JERSEY

AIDS Coalition of Southern New Jersey (formerly the AIDS Resource Coalition)
Northgate Plaza 1
7th and Linden Streets
Camden, NJ 08102
Office: (609) 966-0330

• Services provided include: buddy programs, support groups, financial advocacy, and referrals. Serves Camden, Gloucester, and Burlington Counties.

AIDS Services Expansion Program
Family Planning Association of New Jersey
132 West State Street
Trenton, NJ 08608
Office: (609) 393-8423

• Offers technical assistance, information, and support to family planning agencies throughout New Jersey. Publishes a low-cost monthly newsletter targetting healthcare workers and focusing on women, children, and minority issues in relation to AIDS.

Area Health Education Center (AHEC)
Northgate Plaza 1
7th and Linden Streets
Camden, NJ 08102
Office: (609) 963-AHEC

• Offers: HIV/AIDS trainings and programs, information, training courses on loss and grief, HIV and ethical issues, values clarification, and more. Bilingual educator for Spanish-speaking audiences available. AIDS Resource Directory for New Jersey available.

Blacks Against AIDS
P.O. Box 7732
Atlantic City, NJ 08404
Contact Ava Brown, Director, at (609) 347-1645.

• Offers education and outreach.

Division of Civil Rights
383 West State Street
Trenton, NJ 08625
Office: (609) 292-4605

• Enforces the New Jersey law against discrimination based on "handicap" in employment, housing, and public accomodations. Those with HIV illness or perceived as such are protected under this law. Provides case-by-case guidance and referrals. Locations throughout New Jersey. In Atlantic City, call (609) 441-3100. In Camden, call (609) 757-2850. In Paterson, call (201) 977-4500.

Hyacinth Foundation AIDS Project
211 Livingston Avenue
New Brunswick, NJ 08901
Office: (908) 246-0925
Hotline: (800) 433-0254 (Monday-Friday, 10 am-10pm; Saturday, 10am-1pm)

• Offers: hotline and referral service, education, support groups, buddy services, financial and legal assistance, advocacy, home care, and short-term emergency services. Serves northern two-thirds of New Jersey.

New Jersey Women and AIDS Network
5 Elm Row
New Brunswick, NJ 08901

• Offers: information and materials on women and AIDS, including "Me First! Medical Manifestations of HIV in Women" (see Appendix A).

State of New Jersey Department of Community Affairs
State Office of Legal Services
CN-800 101 South Broad Street
Trenton, NJ 08625
Office: (609) 292-6262

• Provides legal referrals. Spanish spoken.

State of New Jersey Department of Health: AIDS Program
AIDS Education and Prevention Unit, CN 363
363 West State Street
Trenton, NJ 08625-0363
Office: (609) 984-6050
24-hr. AIDS Hotline: (800) 624-2377

• Provides: education, referrals, information, and outreach.

NATIONAL ORGANIZATIONS

Association of Asian/Pacific Community Health Organizations
310 8th Street, Suite 210
Oakland, CA 94607
Office: (415) 272-9536

• Offers information on health programs and materials.

LAMBDA Legal Defense and Education Fund, Inc.
666 Broadway
New York, NY 10012
Office: (212) 995-8585

• A public interest law firm providing legal defense for gay men, lesbians, and PWAs in primarily test case/impact litigation; a newsletter, *AIDS Update*, covering AIDS litigation nation-wide; and education, advocacy, and conferences.

Multicultural Prevention Resources
1540 Market Street, Suite 320
San Francisco, CA 94102
Office: (415) 861-2142

•Provides training, technical assistance, and publications on AIDS for programs serving people of color.

National AIDS Information Clearinghouse
P.O. Box 6003
Rockville, MD 20850
Office: (301) 762-5111

• Offers information and referrals for health professionals, distributes federal AIDS publications, and accesses databases listing agencies and materials.

National Association of People with AIDS
P.O. Box 65472
Washington, DC 20035
Office: (202) 483-7979

• Offers: quarterly newsletter, *NAPWA News*, and a speakers bureau.

National Council of La Raza
AIDS Project
810 First Street, NE, 3rd Floor
Washington, DC 20002
Office: (202) 289-1380

• Seeks to expand AIDS education in the Hispanic community. Works with 80 La Raza affiliates nationwide.

National Native American AIDS Prevention Center
6239 College Avenue, Suite 201
Oakland, CA 94618
Office: (415) 658-2051

• Provides videos and print materials as well as training and technical assistance.

National Resource Center on Women and AIDS
c/o Center for Women Policy Studies
2000 P Street, NW
Suite 508
Washington, DC 20036
Office: (212) 872-1770

• Provides information and resource materials.

National Women's Health Network
1325 G Street, NW, Lower Level
Washington, DC 20005
Office: (202) 347-1140

• Provides publications and referral information on women and AIDS.

Native American Women's Health Education Resource Center
P.O. Box 572
Lake Andes, SD 57356-0572
Office: (605) 487-7072

• Provides pre- and post-test counseling, support groups, prevention workshops, and culturally-specific posters, pamphlets, and videos.

San Francisco AIDS Foundation
Educational and Marketing Division
333 Valencia Street, 4th Floor
San Francisco, CA 94103

OR:
Client Services and Administration
25 Van Ness Avenue
Suite 660
San Francisco, CA 94102
Office: (415) 864-4376

• Provides numerous AIDS educational materials and quarterly catalog.

Sex Information Education Council of the United States (SIECUS)
130 West 42nd Street, Suite 2500
New York, NY 10036
Office: (212) 819-9770

• Offers sex education curricula, a bilingual brochure on how to talk to children about AIDS, an annotated bibliography on AIDS education, a speakers bureau on sex education, and a library.

C

SAMPLE CLIENT NEEDS ASSESSMENT SURVEY

Please see Chapter Two for a discussion of how to use this form.

		YES	NO
1.	Would you like more information about HIV/AIDS?	❑	❑
2.	Would you like to learn more about how people get HIV/AIDS?	❑	❑
3.	Would you like to learn more about HIV/AIDS and giving blood?	❑	❑
4.	Would you like to learn more about HIV/AIDS and safer sex?	❑	❑
5.	Are you interested in learning how to talk to your partner about safer sex?	❑	❑
6.	Do you have questions about dating and safer sex?	❑	❑

7. Do you have other questions about safer sex? What are they? _____
_____
_____

8.	Do you have any questions about HIV/AIDS and drugs?	❑	❑
9.	Would you like to learn more about the HIV (AIDS) Antibody test?	❑	❑
10.	Do you have any questions about birth control and HIV/AIDS?	❑	❑
11.	Do you have any questions about becoming pregnant and HIV/AIDS?	❑	❑
12.	Would you like information about babies with HIV/AIDS?	❑	❑
13.	If you have children, have you ever spoken with them about HIV/AIDS?	❑	❑
13a.	Would you like to meet with other women to discuss how to talk about HIV/AIDS with your children?	❑	❑

13b. Do you have other questions about HIV/AIDS and your children? What are they? _____

_____

_____

14. Do you have any questions about HIV/AIDS on the job? _____

_____

_____

15. Do you ever worry about HIV/AIDS and the health of your family or friends? Please explain:

_____

_____

16. Do you ever worry about HIV/AIDS and your own health? Please explain: _____

_____

_____

16a. Would you like a safe, private place to talk about your concerns?   ☐   ☐

17. Do you have HIV-related disease or HIV infection?   ☐   ☐

17a. If yes, would you like a safe, private place to talk about your concerns?   ☐   ☐

18. Do you have a friend or loved one with HIV-related disease?   ☐   ☐

18a. Would you like a support group to talk about your feelings about   ☐   ☐
     his/her illness?

19. Are you currently caring for someone with HIV/AIDS?   ☐   ☐

19a. Would you like a support group to talk about your feelings or   ☐   ☐
     problems with caring for someone with HIV/AIDS?

20. What other issues (about HIV/AIDS or anything else) would you like more information about?

_____

_____

21. Would you be interested in volunteering some time to work on   ☐   ☐
     services or programs for women or families with HIV/AIDS?

D

SAMPLE COMMUNITY NEEDS ASSESSMENT SURVEY

The following questionnaire is intended to provide information about the programs and services that exist in you community. It is also a tool for identifying gaps in services. The questionnaire highlights the following key areas of concern: services, accessibility and appropriateness, outreach, education, general health service delivery, drug treatment options, HIV antibody testing and counseling, public policy, and special populations. For a discussion of how to implement this survey, see Chapter Two.

Instructions: Answer as many of the questions as you can based on your knowledge of the resources available in your community and the referral resources at your disposal. Use phone interviews or work group meetings to get specific information on how local organizations are meeting the needs of women, and where there are gaps in appropriate services.

A. Does your town/region/district have one or more community-based organizations that either focus exclusively on HIV disease or have some HIV-related component(s)?

B. List all such organizations. If you live in an area with a large number of HIV-related and/or community-based organizations, list only those in your immediate area, or those to which you would be likely to refer your clients.

For each organization you have listed above, answer questions 1-63, adding or deleting questions as appropriate.

SERVICES

1. What kinds of HIV-related services are provided (e.g., education, direct service, information/referral, etc.)? Be specific (e.g., what *kind* of direct services are provided?)

2. What populations are served?

3. What, if any, are their eligibility requirements? (e.g., do they serve only people with CDC-defined AIDS or all people with HIV disease?)

4. Do they serve women? How many women do they currently serve?

5. Of the women they serve, do most have HIV disease or are they primarily partners/friends/parents of people with HIV disease?

6. If the organization offers HIV-related counseling, does it have female counselors?

7. Are all counselors trained to be sensitive to special issues for women (e.g. women's health, reproductive issues, sexual assault, etc.)?

8. Does the organization offer special programs for women? (e.g. women-only support groups, childcare, etc.) If so, what kind?

9. Are services provided for care partners (friends, family members, or partners who take primary responsibility for the care of a person with HIV disease)?

ACCESSIBILITY AND APPROPRIATENESS

10. Is the organization easily accessible by public transportation?

11. Does the organization have a transportation service?

12. Will the organization help pay transportation costs?

13. Are the premises wheelchair-accessible and accessible to physically challenged persons?

14. What are the organization's hours?

15. What, if any, are the evening, weekend, and emergency hours?

16. Does the organization have a hotline/phone machine that provides referrals in emergency situations?

17. Is childcare provided (or paid) for those attending the programs?

18. What languages are spoken by program staff? Do these match those of the women who might want to use the services?

19. Do program staff reflect the cultural groups that will use these services? If not, are they sensitive to these groups? How do they meet the needs of these groups?

OUTREACH

20. Does the organization conduct outreach to women in the community? How is this outreach done?

21. Is outreach to special populations of women undertaken by outreach teams with appropriate language skills and cultural awareness?

22. Are the outreach teams staffed by people who come from or understand the community itself?

EDUCATION

23. Are education and prevention materials (print, audiovisual, etc.) offered by the program?

24. If so, are there materials geared for women?

25. Are the materials on women and HIV accurate and pro-empowerment?

26. Do these materials offer women choices and options regarding reproductive decisions, testing, etc.?

27. Are materials geared for persons of varying educational backgrounds and reading levels?

28. Are outreach materials available in the languages spoken in the community?

29. Are audiovisual materials made available to persons who cannot or do not read?

30. Describe the kinds of general community education currently taking place.

31. Do HIV-related educational programs and presentations for the community always include a component on women?

32. Is any community education geared to women in particular - e.g. by doing HIV education at supermarkets, churches, women's clubs, through day care programs, schools, or in other settings where women might not otherwise be reached with this information?

33. Is there a local library or file of articles, books, and information on women and HIV?

The following are general questions to give you a sense of the range of services and populations served in your area:

HEALTH SERVICE DELIVERY ISSUES

34. Is there a public hospital or clinic in your area?

35. Have the staff at the hospital received training on HIV disease?

36. Have the staff at the hospital received training on women and HIV disease in particular?

37. Are there other low-cost or free health services programs in your area?

38. Do these low-cost or free programs have experience in serving people with HIV?

DRUG TREATMENT OPTIONS

39. What type of drug treatment exists in your area?

40. Is there a waiting list for individuals wishing to go into treatment for drug addiction? If so, how long is the wait?

41. Does the local program accept people with HIV disease?

42. Does the local program accept women?

43. Does it accept pregnant women?

44. Does it accept women and their children?

45. Does the local program provide HIV education for clients?

46. Does the program provide HIV education for the partners and families of clients?

HIV TESTING AND COUNSELING ISSUES

47. Is there an HIV antibody test site* in your region?

48. Is testing done anonymously or confidentially?

49. Does this site offer counseling before offering the test?

49a. What does the counseling session consist of?

49b. Is the counseling non-directive?**

49c. If counseling is not provided beforehand, does the site refer people elsewhere for counseling, or does it simply test people without pre-test counseling?

50. Does the testing site offer post-test counseling?

50a. If so, does it offer follow-up after the first session?

50b. If not, does it refer for post-test counseling?

51. Does it offer ongoing counseling or support groups for people who test HIV positive?

---

* May not be a test site exclusively, but some other type of service organization that provides HIV antibody testing, such as a family planning clinic or health center.

** Non-directive counseling means that a client is provided with accurate information and is presented with options and choices. They are not told what to do or pressured to make a certain decision.

POLICY ISSUES

52. How is local HIV/AIDS policy determined?

53. Are women's advocates in the key decision-making roles or on committee(s) making recommendations on policy and procedures?

54. Do local health or civil rights advocacy organizations address women's issues?

POPULATIONS THAT NEED TO BE REACHED

55. Are there programs reaching out to children with HIV disease and their mothers/families?

56. Are there programs reaching out to incarcerated women?

57. Are there programs reaching out to IV drug users and their partners?

58. Are there programs reaching out to other substance-abusing women?

59. Are there programs reaching out to homeless women?

60. Are there programs reaching out to adolescents?

61. Are there programs reaching out to sex workers?

62. Are there programs reaching out to lesbians?

63. Are the programs reaching out to women in different cultural communities? (If so, by what means? Are there any cultural groups in your area that are not being reached?)

REFERENCES

"Against All Odds: Grassroots Minority Groups Fight AIDS." *Health/PAC Bulletin*. Spring 1988. pp. 4-10.

Ahmann, Sarah. "Patterns of AIDS Spread Elicit Proposals to Tighten Precautions: Special Guidelines for Obstetricians." *Ob. Gyn. News*. Vol. 22, No. 12. July 15-31, 1987. p.1.

"AIDS and Women: The Shadow Lengthens." *New York Daily News*. July 16, 1990.

"AIDS Forecasting: Undercounting of Cases and Lack of Key Data Weaken Existing Estimates." *U.S. General Accounting Office Report to Congressional Requesters*. July 1989.

"AIDS is Reported as No. 9 Cause of Death Among Children 1 to 4." *New York Times*. December 20, 1988. p. A10.

"AIDS Panel Agrees on Sex Counseling of Catholic Patients." *New York Times*. March 2, 1988.

"Alcohol May Hasten Spread of AIDS in Infected People." *New York Times*. May 5, 1988. p. 13.

Alexander, P. *Prostitutes and AIDS: Scapegoating and the Law — An AIDS Information Packet*. San Francisco: National Task Force on Prostitution. 1988. 32 pages.

Alexander, P. *Prostitutes Prevent AIDS: A Manual for Health Educators*. San Francisco: California Prostitutes Education Program. 1988.

Altman, Lawrence K. "Antibodies Seem to Protect Fetus from AIDS." *New York Times*. May 1, 1990. p. B9.

Altman, Lawrence K. "Communicable Diseases Masked Behind Doctors' Erratic Reporting." *New York Times*. July 10, 1990. p. C3.

Altman, Lawrence K. "Who's Stricken and How: AIDS Pattern is Shifting." *New York Times*. February 5, 1989. p. A1.

Amaro, Hortensia. "Hispanic Women and AIDS: Considerations for Prevention and Research." *Psychology of Women Quarterly*. 1988;12. pp. 429-43.

Amaro, Hortensia. "Women's Reproductive Rights in the Age of AIDS: New Threats to Informed Choice." Presented at the Division of the Psychology of Women at the 97th Annual Convention of the American Psychological Association, New Orleans, LA. August 11-15, 1989.

American Bar Association AIDS Coordinating Committee. *AIDS: The Legal Issues*. Washington, DC. 1988. 252 pages.

American Foundation for AIDS Research. *Learning AIDS: An Information Resources Directory, Second Edition*. New York: R.R. Bowker. 1989.

Andriote, JM, and Medina, V. "For Women at Risk, Prevention Begins with Self-Esteem." *The National AIDS Network (NAN) Monitor*. Fall 1988. Volume 3, No. 1. pp. 12-15.

Angier, Natalie. "Americans' Sex Knowledge is Lacking, Poll Says." *New York Times*. September 6, 1990.

Bakeman, R, et al. "The Incidence of AIDS Among Blacks and Hispanics." *Journal of the National Medical Association*. 1987;79. pp. 921-8.

Baker, JN, et al. "Learning to Live with AIDS in Prisons." *New York Newsweek*. February 13, 1989. pp. 27-8.

Bell, NK. "AIDS and Women: Remaining Ethical Issues." *AIDS Education and Prevention*. 1989;1(1). pp. 22-30.

"Bias in Research." From the Los Angeles Times. *New York Newsday*. August 28, 1990.

Bishop, Jerry E. "AIDS Set to Be a Leading Killer of Women in '91." *Wall Street Journal*. July 11, 1990.

Bishop, Katherine. "Prostitute in Jail after AIDS Report." *New York Times*. July 15, 1990.

Brown, LS, Jr., and Primm, BJ. "Intravenous Drug Abuse and AIDS in Minorities." *AIDS Public Policy Journal*. 1988;3(2). pp. 5-15.

Brownworth, Victoria A. "HIV Testing, Rape Survivors and the Law." *Outweek*. October 31, 1990. p. 12.

Buckingham, Stephan L, and Rehm, Susan. "AIDS and Women at Risk." *Health and Social Work*. Winter 1987. pp. 5-11.

Campbell, Carole A. "Women and AIDS." *Social Science Medicine*. Vol. 30, No. 4. 1990. pp. 407-15.

Carper, Alison. "Abortion Seekers Face AIDS Bias." *New York Newsday*. October 23, 1990.

Case, P, et al. The Social Context of AIDS Risk Behavior among Intravenous Drug-Using Lesbians in San Francisco. Presented at the IV International Conference on AIDS, June 12-16, 1988. Stockholm, Sweden (unpublished).

Center for Population Options (CPO). *The Facts: Adolescents, AIDS, and Human Immunodeficiency Virus*. Washington, DC: Center for Population Options. 1989.

Centers for Disease Control. "AIDS Weekly Surveillance Report — United States." Weekly publication.

Chu, Susan Y, et al. "Epidemiology of Reported Cases of AIDS in Lesbians, United States 1980-89." *American Journal of Public Health*. November 1990. Vol. 80, No. 11.

Cimons, Marlene. "Children's Drug Trials Come of Age amid AIDS Epidemic." *Staten Island Advance*. August 21, 1990. p. A7.

Cimons, Marlene. "For Women, AIDS Brings Special Woes." *Los Angeles Times*. January 8, 1988.

Coates, TJ, et al. "AIDS Antibody Testing: Will It Stop the AIDS Epidemic? Will It Help People Infected with HIV?" *American Psychology*. 1988;43(11). pp. 859-64.

Cohen, J, et al. "Prostitutes and AIDS: Public Policy Issues." *AIDS Public Policy Journal*. 1988;3(2). pp. 16-22.

Colasanto, D. "Public Still Holds Faulty AIDS Beliefs." *San Francisco Chronicle*. November 29, 1989. p. A5.

Colen, BD. "Heterosexual AIDS: Truth v. Myth." *New York Newsday*. February 27, 1990.

Collins, Janet L, and Britton, Patti O. *Training Educators in HIV Prevention: An Inservice Manual*. Network Publications, Santa Cruz, CA. 1990.

Communication Technologies and Research and Decisions Corp. *Reaching Ethnic Communities in the Fight Against AIDS*. August 1, 1986. For the San Francisco AIDS Foundation, San Francisco.

COSSMHO (National Coalition of Hispanic Health and Human Services Organizations). *AIDS Service Directory for Hispanics*. 1030 15th Street, N.W., Suite 1053, Washington, DC 20005. April 1987.

Delacoste, F, and Alexander, P (eds). *Sex Work: Writings by Women in the Sex Industry*. Pittsburgh, PA: Cleis Press. 1988. 349 pages.

De La Rosa, M. "Health Care Needs of Hispanic Americans and the Responsiveness of the Health Care System." *Health Social Work*. 1989;14(2). pp. 104-13.

De La Vega, Ernesto. "Considerations for Reaching the Latino Population with Sexuality and HIV/AIDS Information and Education." *Sex Information Education Council of the United States (SIECUS) Report*. Feb/March 1990. Vol. 18. No. 3.

Denenberg, Risa. "Toward a Lesbian Health Agenda." *Outweek*. August 8, 1990.

Denenberg, Risa. "Women and HIV-Related Conditions." *Treatment and Research Forum*. Community Research Initiative. October 1990.

Des Jarlais, DC, and Friedman, SR. "Intravenous Cocaine, Crack, and HIV Infection." *Journal of the American Medical Association.* 1988;259. pp. 1945-6.

Des Jarlais, DC, and Friedman, SR. "Target Groups for Preventing AIDS among Intravenous Drug Users." *Journal of Applied Psychology.* 1987;17(3). pp. 251-68.

DiClemente, RJ, et al. "Minorities and AIDS: Knowledge, Attitudes and Misconceptions among Black and Latino Adolescents." *American Journal of Public Health.* 1988;78. pp. 55-7.

DiClemente, RJ. "Prevention of Human Immunodeficiency Virus Infection among Adolescents: The Interplay of Health Education and Public Policy in the Development and Implementation of School-Based AIDS Education Programs." *AIDS Education and Prevention.* 1989;1(1). pp. 70-8.

Dobie, D. "An Interview with Yolanda Serrano." *Ms.* January/February 1989. pp. 79-83.

Dolman, Cathy. "AIDS' Attack on Teens." *New York Newsday.* June 15, 1990.

Donovan, P. "AIDS and Family Planning Clinics: Confronting the Crisis." *Family Planning Perspectives.* 1987;19. pp. 111-4, 138.

Easthope, Tracey, and Asetoyer, Charon. "The Impact of AIDS in the Native American Community." Native American Women's Health Education Resource Center, a Project of the Native American Community Board, P.O. Box 572, Lake Andes, SD 57356-0572. 1988. 43 pages.

Eskenazi, B, et al. "HIV Serology in Artificially Inseminated Lesbians." *Journal of AIDS.* 1989;2. pp. 187-93.

Evans, Heidi. "HIV Tied to Cervix Cancer." *New York Daily News.* April 29, 1990.

Fischl, MA, et al. "Evaluation of Heterosexual Partners, Children, and Household Contacts of Adults with AIDS." *Journal of the American Medical Association.* 1987; 257. pp. 640-4.

"Forty-four percent of Doctors Report Tests for AIDS on Donated Semen." *New York Times.* August 11, 1988. p. 15.

Freudenberg, N, et al. "How Black and Latino Community Organizations Respond to the AIDS Epidemic: A Case Study in One New York City Neighborhood." *AIDS Education and Prevention.* 1989;1(1). pp. 12-21.

Friedland, GH, and Klein, RS. "Transmission of the Human Immunodeficiency Virus." *New England Journal of Medicine.* 1987;317. pp. 1125-35.

Garrett, Laurie. "Three Reports Study Pregnancy, AIDS." *New York Newsday.* March 3, 1989. p. 15.

Garrett, Laurie. "Women's Unexplained Deaths Cited." *New York Newsday.* June 14, 1988. p. 9.

Garrett, Laurie. "World Health Group: AIDS Spreading Faster." *New York Newsday.* June 13, 1990.

Gee, Gayling, and Moran, Theresa A (eds). *AIDS: Concepts in Nursing Practice*. Baltimore: Williams & Wilkins. 1988.

Glaberson, William. "Fear of AIDS with Rape: How a Case was Affected." *New York Times*. July 9, 1990. p. A16.

Goleman, Daniel. "Lies Men Tell Put Women in Danger of AIDS." *New York Times*. August 14, 1988. p. 29.

Gordon, Shirley. "Plight in New York." Letter to the Editor. *New York Times*. September 12, 1990.

Greif, GL, and Porembski, E. "Significant Others of IV Drug Abusers with AIDS: New Challenges for Drug Treatment Programs." *Journal of Substance Abuse Treatment*. 1987;4. pp. 151-5.

Guinan, ME, and Hardy, A. "Women and AIDS: The Future is Grim." *Journal of the American Medical Women's Association*. 1987;42. pp. 157-8.

Haffner, Debra W. "AIDS and Adolescents: School Health Education Must Begin Now." *Journal of School Health*. April 1988, Vol. 58, No. 4. p. 154.

Hamilton, Jean, and Sparks, Caroline H. *Protection Against Infection for Women Using Alternative Insemination*. The Feminist Institute Clearinghouse, P.O. Box 30563, Bethesda, MD 20814. 1988.

Hilts, Philip J. "AIDS Panel Finds U.S. Failure in Providing Care." *New York Times*. December 7, 1989.

Hilts, Philip J. "Bush, in First Address on AIDS, Backs a Bill to Protect Its Victims." *New York Times*. March 30, 1990. p. A1.

Hilts, Philip J. "Spread of AIDS by Heterosexuals Remains Slow." *New York Times*. May 1, 1990. p. B5.

"HIV-Related Beliefs, Knowledge, and Behaviors among High School Students." Reprinted by the U.S. Department of Health and Human Services, Public Health Service from *Morbidity Mortality Weekly Review*. December 2, 1988. Vol. 37, No. 47. pp. 717-721.

Hoff, R, et al. "Seroprevalence of Human Immunodeficiency Virus among Childbearing Women." *New England Journal of Medicine*. 1988;318(9). pp. 525-30.

International Working Group on Women and AIDS. *An Open Letter to the Planning Committees of the International Conference on AIDS*. San Francisco Women in AIDS. Undated.

Isaacs, Rebecca. "Women and AIDS." Interview with Ruth Schwartz. *The Exchange*. National Lawyers Guild AIDS Network, 211 Gough Street, Third Floor, San Francisco, CA 94102. Issue 7, 1988.

Johnson, Dirk. "AIDS Clamor at Colleges Muffling Older Dangers." *New York Times*. March 8, 1990.

Kiefer, Renata. "Issues in Pediatric AIDS and HIV Infection." *Multicultural Inquiry and Research on AIDS (MIRA).* Vol. 4, No.3. September 1990. p. 1.

Kolata, Gina. "AIDS is Killing Women Faster, Researchers Say." *New York Times.* October 19, 1987. p. A1.

Kolata, Gina. "Experts Say Women at Risk are Well-Informed on AIDS." *New York Times.* September 30, 1987. p. 10.

Kolata, Gina. "How to Ask about Sex and Get Honest Answers." *Science.* 1988;230. p. 382.

Kolder, Veronika EB, et al. "Court Ordered Obstetrical Interventions." *New England Journal of Medicine.* Special Article. May 7, 1987. pp. 1192-6.

Kranes, Marsha. "Poll: Many Women Think AIDS Hits Only Gays." *New York Post.* December 12, 1989.

Lambert, Bruce. "AIDS Deaths Near Another Awful Record." *New York Times.* March 25, 1990. p. E20.

Lambert, Bruce. "AIDS in Black Women Seen as Leading Killer." *New York Times.* July 11, 1990. p. A14.

Lambert, Bruce. "AIDS Legacy: A Growing Generation of Orphans." *New York Times.* July 17, 1989. p. A1.

Lambert, Bruce. "As AIDS Spreads, So Do Warnings for Partners." *New York Times.* May 15, 1990.

Lambert, Bruce. "Autopsy Tests for AIDS Find 1 in 7 Infected." *New York Times.* August 30, 1990. p. A20.

Lambert, Bruce. "Doctors Urged to Counsel All about AIDS." *New York Times.* March 2, 1990. p. A13.

La Rosa, Paul. "Women and AIDS: In Study, 94% Say They'd Tell if They Had It." *New York Daily News.* December 12, 1989.

Leary, Warren E. "Gloomy Report on the Health of Teen-Agers." *New York Times.* June 9, 1990.

Lee, DA, and Fong, K. "HIV/AIDS and the Asian and Pacific Islander Community." *Sex Information Education Council of the United States (SIECUS) Report.* Vol. 18. No. 3. February/March 1990.

Lee, Felicia R. "Black Doctors Urge Study of Factors in Risk of AIDS." *New York Times.* July 21, 1989. p. B7.

Lemp, GF, et al. "Survival Trends for Patients with AIDS." *Journal of the American Medical Association.* 263(3). 1990.

"Life Expectancy Rates Widen Over Racial Lines." *New York Times.* March 16, 1989. p. B9.

Macks, Judy. "Countertransference Reactions of Female Health Care Providers to Women with HIV Infections." *Focus: A Guide to AIDS Research and Counseling.* March 1988. pp. 3.

Macks, Judy. "Women and AIDS: Countertransference Issues. *Social Casework: The Journal of Contemporary Social Work.* 1988. p.340.

Marmor, M, et al. "Possible Female-to-Female Transmission of Human Immunodeficiency Virus" (letter). *Annals of Internal Medicine.* 1986;105(6). p. 969.

Martin, A Damien. "Learning to Hide: The Socialization of the Gay Adolescent." *Adolescent Psychiatry: Developmental and Clinical Studies.* Vol. X. University of Chicago. 1982.

Mayfield, Mark. "AIDS Cases Surge in Non-Urban Areas." *USA Today.* September 13, 1990.

Mays, VM, and Cochran, SD. "Issues in the Perception of AIDS Risk and Risk Reduction Activities by Black and Hispanic/Latina Women." *American Psychology.* 1988;43. pp. 949-57.

McCarthy, Sheryl. "Of Abortions, Fear of AIDS and Surgery on the Psyche." *New York Newsday.* October 24, 1990.

McFadden, Laura K. "A Woman's Protection." *New York Newsday.* July 24, 1990.

Medina, C. "Latino Culture and Sex Education." *Sex Information and Education Council of the United States (SIECUS) Report,* January-February 1987. pp. 1-4.

Minkoff, HL. "Care of Pregnant Women Infected with Human Immunodeficiency Virus." *Journal of the American Medical Association.* 1987;258. pp. 2714-7.

Minkowitz, D. "Safe and Sappho: An AIDS Primer for Lesbians." *The Village Voice.* February 21, 1989. p. 21.

Mitchell, Janet. "What about the Mothers of HIV-Infected Babies?" *National AIDS Network (NAN) Multi-Cultural Notes on AIDS Education and Service.* April 1988. Volume1, No. 10. pp. 2-3.

Mitchell, Janet. "Women, AIDS, and Public Policy." *AIDS Public Policy Journal* 1988;3(2). pp. 50-2.

Mondanaro, Josette. *Chemically Dependent Women: Assessment and Treatment.* Lexington, MA: DC Heath and Company. 1989. 170 pages.

Mondanaro, Josette. "Strategies for AIDS Prevention: Motivating Health Behavior in Drug Dependent Women." *Journal of Psychoactive Drugs.* April-June 1987. Vol. 19(2). pp. 99-105.

Monzon, OT, and Capellan, JMB. "Female-to-Female Transmission of HIV" (letter). *Lancet.* 1987;8549(2). pp. 40-1.

Mujeres en Acción Pro Salud Reproductiva: Northeast Project on Latina Women and Reproductive Health and Women of Color Partnership Program RCAR Educational Fund. *Puertorriqueñas: Sociodemographics, Health and Reproductive Issues Among Puerto Rican Women in the U.S.* Hispanic Health Council, 98 Cedar Street, 3-A, Hartford, CT 06106.

Muller C. "Medicaid: The Lower Tier of Health Care for Women." *Women and Health.* 1988;14(2). pp. 81-103.

National Indian Health Board, "AIDS in Indian Country: Caution, Health Education and Prevention Seen as Key to Controlling Spread of Virus." *National Indian Health Board Reporter.* October 1987. p. 12-20.

New Hampshire Coalition Against Domestic and Sexual Violence. *Position Paper on HIV Testing of Sexual Assault Victim/Survivors.* P.O. Box 353, Concord, NH 03301.

New York City AIDS Fund. *AIDS, Community Needs and Private Funding: A Needs Assessment for New York City.* October 1988.

New York City Commission on Human Rights. "Women and AIDS — A Report." AIDS Discrimination Unit." 1987.

New York City Department of Health. *HIV Serosurvey Report* on seroprevalence of HIV infection among adolescents in New York City. Vol. 1. No. 2. July 1990.

New York State Department of Health. *A Physician's Guide to HIV Counseling and Testing of Women of Childbearing Age.* Albany: New York State Department of Health. 1988.

New York State Department of Health. *Focus on AIDS in New York State.* Newsletter of the NYS Department of Health. Issue on Women and the Impact of the HIV/AIDS Epidemic. Vol. 2. No. 2. October 1990.

New York State Women's Division. *Women and AIDS Project Newsletter.* Albany, NY.

Newman, Anthony. "Patterns of AIDS Spread Elicit Proposals to Tighten Precautions: Involuntary Sterilizations?" *Ob.Gyn.News.* Vol. 22, No. 12. July 15-31, 1987.

Newman, Robert, et al. "Report and Recommendations Regarding Exposure to HIV through Rape and Occupational Injury." AIDS Advisory Council Subcommittee on Occupational Issues. January 11, 1990.

Nissley, Barbara A. *Acquired Immune Deficiency Syndrome and Victims of Sexual Violence.* Policy Issue Paper #3. Pennsylvania Coalition Against Rape. August 1988.

Norwood, Chris. "Alarming Risk in Deaths: Are Women Showing New AIDS Symptoms?" *Ms.* July 1988. pp. 65-7.

NOVA Research Company. *Conference on AIDS Intervention Strategies for Female Sexual Partners.*

Volume 1. June 1989.

NOVA Research Company, National Institute on Drug Abuse (NIDA) Community Research Branch. *Conference on AIDS Intervention Strategies for Female Sexual Partners: Sexual Partner Program Descriptions*. Volume 2. June 1989.

NOVA Research Company, National Institute on Drug Abuse (NIDA) Community Research Branch. *Women and AIDS: An Annotated Bibliography*. May 1990. NOVA, 4600 East-West Highway, Suite 700, Bethesda, MD 20814.

Nze, R, et al. "Supporting the mother and infant at risk for AIDS." *Nursing*. 1987;17. pp. 44-7.

Osterholm, MT, and MacDonald, KL. "Facing the Complex Issues of Pediatric AIDS: A Public Health Perspective" (editorial). *Journal of the American Medical Association*. 1987;258. pp. 2736-7.

Patton, C, and Kelly, J. *Making It—A Woman's Guide to Sex in the Age of AIDS*. Ithaca, NY: Firebrand Books, 141 The Commons, Ithaca, NY 14850. 1987. 53 pages. $3.95.

Potler, Cathy. *AIDS in Prison: A Crisis in New York State Corrections*. The Correctional Association of New York. June 1988.

Purvis, Andrew. "Research for Men Only." *Time*. March 5, 1990.

"Red Cross Fails to Note Possible AIDS-Tied Blood." *Wall Street Journal*. July 11, 1990.

Richardson, Diane. *Women and AIDS*. New York: Methuen, Inc., 1988.

Rickert, Vaughn I, et al. "Adolescents and AIDS: Females Attitudes and Behaviors Toward Condom Purchase and Use." Society for Adolescent Medicine. 1989. Elsevier Science Publishing Co., Inc. New York. p. 313.

Rieder, I, and Ruppelt, P (eds). *AIDS: The Women*. Pittsburgh, PA: Cleis Press, 1988.

Rosenthal, Elisabeth. "Abortion Clinics Often Reject Patients With the AIDS Virus." *New York Times*. October 23, 1990. p. A15.

Rosenthal, Elisabeth. "The Spread of AIDS: A Mystery Unravels." *New York Times*. August 28, 1990. p. B5.

Rothenberg, R, et al. "Survival with the Acquired Immunodeficiency Syndrome." *New England Journal of Medicine*. 317(21). 1987. pp. 1297-1302.

Rowell, Ron. "Native Americans: Historic Problems Hamper AIDS Prevention and Care." *National AIDS Network (NAN) Multi-Cultural Notes on AIDS Education and Service*. May 1988. Volume 1, No. 11. pp. 1-3.

Rowell, Ron. "Native Americans, Stereotypes, and HIV/AIDS." *Sex Information Education Council of the United States (SIECUS) Report.* Vol. 18. No. 3. February/March 1990

Sachs, BP, et al. "Acquired Immunodeficiency Syndrome: Suggested Protocol for Counseling and Screening in Pregnancy." *Obstet Gynecol.* 1987;70. pp. 408-11.

Salholz, Eloise, et al. "A Frightening Aftermath: Concern About AIDS Adds to the Trauma of Rape." *New York Newsweek.* July 23, 1990. p. 53.

Schmich, MT. "Women and AIDS: The Hidden Toll — Forgotten Victims of Disease Face Lonely Deaths." *Chicago Tribune.* June 4, 1989. Section 1, pp. 1,20.

Schulman, Sarah. "Women Need Not Apply: Institutional Discrimination in AIDS Drug Trials." *The Village Voice.*

Selwyn, Peter A, et al. "Knowledge of HIV Antibody Status and Decisions to Continue or Terminate Pregnancy among Intravenous Drug Users." *Journal of the American Medical Association.* June 23/ 30, 1989.

Selwyn, Peter A, et al. "Prospective Study of Human Immundeficiency Virus Infection and Pregnancy Outcomes in Intravenous Drug Users." *Journal of the American Medical Association.* March 3, 1989;261(9). pp. 1289-94.

Shaw, Nancy. "Model Programs for Women's AIDS Education & Services." San Francisco AIDS Foundation. November 20, 1985.

Shaw, Nancy. Preventing AIDS among Women: The Role of Community Organizing. *Socialist Review.* Fall 1988. pp. 77-92.

Shaw, Nancy, and Paleo, Lyn. "Women and AIDS." *What to do About AIDS.* Leon McKusick (ed.). Berkeley: University of California Press. 1986. pp. 143-53.

Slaughter, Ruth. "Responding to the AIDS Crisis: The Challenge to Shelters." *The Exchange.* Vol. 3, No. 1. Fall/Winter 1988-89.

Smith, Kimberleigh J. "AIDS: A No. 1 Problem for Women of Color." *The City Sun.* August 1-7, 1990.

Smothers, Ronald. "Spread of AIDS in Rural Areas Testing Georgia." *New York Times.* April 18, 1990. p. A8.

Sociomedical Resource Association, Inc. "Safety Guide for the Working Girl" (pamphlet). Sociomedical Resource Association, Inc., 181 Post Road West, Westport, CT 06990. 1988. 12 pages.

Stein, Loren, and Mistiaen, Veronique. "Pregnant in Prison." *The Progressive.* February 1988. pp. 18-21.

Stein, Zena A. "HIV Prevention: The Need for Methods Women Can Use." *American Journal of Public Health.* 0090-0036/90. 1990. p. 460.

"Students Found to Lack AIDS Facts." *New York Newsday*. June 15, 1990.

United States Department of Health and Human Services, Department of Agriculture. *Cross Cultural Counseling: A Guide for Nutrition and Health Counselors*.

United States Department of Health and Human Services, Public Health Service. *Report of the Surgeon General's Workshop on Children with HIV Infection and their Families*. Rockville, MD. 1987. (DHHS Publication No. HRS-D-MC 87-1).

Vermund, Sten H, et al. "Acquired Immunodeficiency Syndrome Among Adolescents: Case Surveillance Profiles in New York City and the Rest of the United States." *American Journal of Diseases of Children*. October 1989. Volume 143. 1989. pp. 1220-1225.

Vrazo, Fawn. "In the Works, a Female Condom." *New York Daily News*. January 22, 1990.

Wharton, Carla L. *AIDS In The Black Community*. New York Urban League Black Papers. Undated.

"What Science Knows About AIDS." *Scientific American*. Volume 259. No. 4. October 1988.

Whyte, J. "Teaching Safe Sex." (letter). *New England Journal of Medicine*. 1988;318. p. 387.

Wilson, Susan N. "Sex Education Declines, Teen-Age Births Rise." Letter to the Editor. *New York Times*. September 12, 1990.

Wofsy, CB. "AIDS and Prostitution." In: Schnazi, RF, and Nahmias, AJ (eds). *AIDS in Children, Adolescents, and Heterosexuals*. New York: Elsevier Science Publishing Company. 1988. pp. 168-9.

Wofsy, CB. "Human Immunodeficiency Virus Infection in Women" (editorial). *Journal of the American Medical Association*. 1987;257. pp. 2074-5.

"Woman Charges Malpractice in Lawsuit on AIDS." *New York Times*. September 23, 1987. p. A17.

Woodard, Catherine. "AIDS Stats Bad News for Women." *New York Newsday*. July 11, 1990.

Woodard, Catherine. "Minority AIDS Rates Higher." *New York Newsday*. August 30, 1990.

Woodard, Catherine. "Prenatal HIV Tests are Urged." *New York Newsday*. March 1, 1990.

Worth, Dooley. "Sexual Decision-Making and AIDS: Why Condom Promotion among Vulnerable Women is Likely to Fail." *Studies in Family Planning*. 20(6). Nov/Dec 1989.

Worth, Dooley, and Rodriguez, R. "Latina Women and AIDS." *Sex Information Education Council of the United States (SIECUS) Report*. January-February 1987. pp. 5-7.

INDEX

About the Author

Gerry Pearlberg developed and directed the Women's Centers and AIDS Project at Women's Action Alliance from 1987 to 1989. She is currently the Coordinator of Funding Initiatives for the Bureau of HIV Program Services at the New York City Department of Health. She lives in Brooklyn.